RAEYAN GOFF

UNLEASH YOUR INNER LIGHT

A WOMAN'S GUIDE TO MENTAL WELLNESS AND FULFILLMENT

ISBN: 978-1-966798-09-5

Table of Contents

A Note From The Author

As women, we often find ourselves pulled in myriad directions, striving to meet external standards of success and perfection. Yet, in this pursuit, we sometimes lose sight of the most important journey of all – the journey inward.

"Radiate" is more than just a book; it is an invitation to rediscover the radiant source of strength and wisdom that lies at the core of our being. It's an exploration of what it means to embrace our inner light and cultivate a profound sense of mental wellness and fulfillment.

Throughout the pages of this book, we'll embark on a transformative voyage together. We'll delve into the depths of self-awareness, compassion, and resilience, uncovering the tools and insights needed to navigate life's challenges with grace and authenticity. I'll share my journey towards self-development, so that you know you're not alone.

But "Radiate" is not merely a guide; it's a celebration of the unique journey each of us undertakes in reclaiming our inner radiance. It's a testament to the power of sisterhood, resilience, and self-discovery.

As we journey together through these chapters, I pray that you feel empowered to honor your truth, embrace your vulnerabilities, and shine brightly in the world. May God allow you the ability to recognize that your light is not a dim flicker but a radiant beacon, capable of illuminating even the darkest of paths.

So, my dear reader, I invite you to open your heart and mind to the transformative possibilities that lie within. Let us embark on this journey of self-discovery and empowerment together, for in the depths of our souls, we find the truest reflections of our strength and resilience, and are able to radiate insight.

Welcome to "Radiate: Unleashing Your Inner Light."
With love and light,

Rae ♡

Every one of us has an inner light—a radiant force waiting to shine brightly in the world. But for many of us, life's trials, doubts, and expectations have dimmed that light, leaving us feeling disconnected from our true selves. I know this feeling because I've been there too.

I wrote Radiate: Unleash Your Inner Light for the woman who feels stuck, the woman who knows she's destined for more but isn't sure how to get there. This book isn't just about inspiring you—it's about guiding you through the real work of self-reflection, healing, and intentional growth.

Through my personal experiences, the lessons I've learned, and the tools I've gathered, I want to show you that you already have everything you need within you. You are worthy, capable, and powerful beyond measure. All you need to do is allow yourself to radiate.

This journey won't be easy, but it will be transformative. Together, we'll break through limiting beliefs, step into your authenticity, and build a life that reflects your highest potential.

Introduction: Not Just Another Self-Help Book

In a world that often asks too much of women, where the pressure to excel in every role – whether as a mother, a wife/partner, employee, or employer, or even as an individual – can become overwhelming, it's crucial to take a step back and focus on what truly matters: your mental health and finding your overarching purpose. As a mental health professional and life coach, I believe that you can most definitely, without a doubt have multiple passions and even multiple purpose in life, however, your overarching purpose is the way that you connect it all and create balance and harmony amid a chaotic world. For me, my overarching purpose is helping women find their purpose in life and achieve fulfillment with their life's circumstance. But I have many sub-purposes and areas of passion for how I plan to accomplish this – businesses, coaching, therapy, writing books, digital products, courses, a blog – the list goes on and on, yet everything is fueled by my desire to help women break generational curses and create their own reality.

When I first came up with the idea of writing a self-help book, I got discouraged and started second guessing myself, as many of us do when we contemplate doing something new. There are thousands of amazing self-help books already out there, 100 or so of which I've already read, I told myself. Is it necessary for you to write another one? There is absolutely an array of self-help books already out there, yet most of them are written by males, and there's nothing wrong with that.

I also know that there's definitely are self-help books out there written by women, but I have not yet found a self-help book that was unique in the information it offered. Most books also aren't written by a black woman, who is currently in her 20's as a single mother. I have a unique narrative of working through my depression and anxiety while counseling and coaching other women on how to get over their own limiting beliefs, struggling with imposter syndrome on a daily basis despite everyone telling me I've made it. My experience is real and raw, written while on the journey instead of afterwards, with actionable steps after each chapter. The only book that comes close to this, is "Year of Yes", the amazing read by Shonda Rhimes that all mothers should read. Although I am a therapist by profession, I am writing this book mostly in the perspective of a coach.

They need this, I told myself. The world needs to hear your story, told your way, in your voice, but most importantly, YOU need this. What's the biggest and fastest way to overcome imposter syndrome? By proving yourself wrong.

Writing my book and telling my story means that there is no way that I can continue to tell myself I don't belong in the rooms that I am currently in and that I don't deserve the opportunities God is affording me. The proof is in the pudding. People don't just write books, help create fulfillment in the lives of hundreds of people through 3 different programs, break generational curses and create generational wealth for current, past, and future generations, and achieve financial freedom as a single mother all before the age of 30 and not be deserving or worthy of it all. At least, it's not an everyday thing, I won't say it's impossible, so I told myself that writing this book was me giving myself my flowers.

A client I had in December of 2023 was telling me how she could see that even with all I had accomplished at the time that I didn't see how I was deserving of every bit of it. I silently agreed because every time anyone would ask me about my credentials and I'd say, "I'm 25 with a master's degree and that I am in school for another masters", they would be shocked and impressed. For me though, it was nothing special and I felt unworthy and uncomfortable with receiving praise. It's like I did it, but I didn't want to take credit for it.

Think of being able to buy a car outright in full or reached a huge milestone in life, but when people ask you about it, you're like "I should have done it faster" or "I could've done more", and you'd rather everyone just move on without acknowledging it. Crazy right?

Well, that was my thinking. At that time, I was about a year into taking my self-development journey and spiritual journey seriously and actually putting a goal behind it to heal and become my truest self. This book goes through exactly what that journey looked like for me in real time, and how I finally decided to walk into and fully unleash my inner light, accepting me and everything that I come with, good, bad, or indifferent.

Radiating is a word I chose to use to describe this transition for several reasons, but I'll just share one with you for now. In college, I was working a student job at UNLV (the University of Nevada, Las Vegas) called UNLVolunteers as a program coordinator. I was in the office on the 3rd floor of the Student Union one day introducing myself to the supervisor of the LEAD Team, a similar student-led program. I told her my name, then said "but you can call me Rae". Rae actually means "ray of light". But I didn't know that at the time. Funny how we've come full circle with it.

She said, "Oh that's cute. Ray, like ray of sunshine. I like it."

At that time, I was at the height of struggling with my mental health and I felt like no one's ray of sunshine, definitely not my own. "Yeah, exactly like that, except it's spelled R-a-e," I stated.

"That fits you."

This conversation was a defining moment for me because after that day, I introduced myself as "Rae, you know like a ray of sunshine, just spelled with an e", all the while not ever truly believing it. But by the end of this book, you will see that I found the confidence in myself, to not only be that "Rae of sunshine" for myself, but also to radiate my light over others until they were able to find their own.

Although I don't consider this book to be about spirituality, I cannot tell my story without bringing my relationship with God into it. It definitely had a lot to do with my self-development journey, because as I grew in my faith, my morals and boundaries also grew naturally. I don't think I could have became my dream woman, and the highest version of myself without God.

By the end of this book, I'm praying you have started to become your own ray of sunshine and can radiate in your own inner light. If you'd like more personalized tips and to receive 1-to-1 coaching sessions, check out uniquetransfhermations.com for a free discovery session. Enjoy the book and enjoy your journey towards self-healing.

Chapter 1: Unveiling the Darkness

Mental illness has always been a silent struggle for many individuals across all age ranges and demographics, but the issue is only progressively getting worse. In fact in one of its articles, the CDC states that "mental illnesses are among the most common health conditions in the United States". CDC Statistics show that there are more than 1 in 5 adults who live with a mental illness, and I am one of them. There are also at least "1 in 5 youth (ages 13-18) either currently or at some point during their life, have had a seriously debilitating mental illness". I was also a part of that statistic, but I had not yet been diagnosed. Later in the chapter we will talk more about the stigma of mental health in the black community. Before we do, take a second to think about your own mental health and that of those around you. How hard it has been to suffer in silence and how anyone around you could be struggling under your nose.

As we set out on this journey together, I invite you to explore the intricacies of our shared experiences but also to be honest with yourself about your own struggles and biases regarding mental health that might not be mentioned here, because we all have them. Think about those moments when life's challenges cast shadows over your ideas of your capabilities: doubts and attitudes created about your strengths, weaknesses, and place in life, how you should/shouldn't act and react to situations, managing stress, and overcoming adversity. These shadows are not always our own and are largely formed based on the ideas we learn from our patriarchal society. Shadows that can take many forms, from the weight of societal expectations to the persistent stigma surrounding mental health. However, within these very shadows, there lies an extraordinary potential for growth and transformation. In this chapter, we embark on a path towards self-discovery, strength, and resilience on the pursuit of mental wellness and fulfillment.

Throughout this chapter, we'll delve into the multifaceted nature of such challenges. We'll begin by celebrating the resilience that defines black women (which we will also expand on within chapter 2, as well as the resilience of women as a whole), acknowledging strengths of this group of women, and drawing inspiration for their triumphs. We will then shine a light on the mental health crisis that affects women across the spectrum. Diving even deeper, we'll unveil the intricate intersectionality of identity from a black woman's perspective, particularly how race and gender intersect in mental health experiences.

In doing so, we cannot ignore the burdens that society places on us as women, insisting that we appear eternally strong and unwavering. We will confront the expectations of perpetual resilience, recognizing the toll it can take on a person's wellbeing, and then using it as a framework to rewrite and tell our own stories.

Each subsection will include a culmination of personal narrative as well as research, coaching, and therapeutic experiences and end with a quiz or other actional step to help you draw parallels between that topic and your own personal experience. Yet, this journey is not all about darkness and healing; it is also about finding the light within and focusing on the positive aspects of your life, a perspective typically known as "living in the and". As we navigate these challenges, I will provide guidance, tools, and strategies for building resilience. I will emphasize the importance of breaking down the stigma surrounding mental health, creating open dialogues with loved ones, and seeking support for your wellbeing without shame.

Ultimately, this chapter serves as the first reminder (of many) that within the darkness, we can uncover the radiant beauty that has been within us all along. So, let's begin this exploration of resilience, self-discovery, and the radiant strength that lies beneath the surface.

Celebrating Resilience: The Strength of a Black Woman

Imagine the bustling streets of New York City, where people rush by, minding their business, without a care in the world for anyone else and their situation. Among them is Michelle, a Black woman who, despite facing formidable challenges, embodies the kindness and grace that most people in today's society lacks. During her job as a housekeeper at a high-end hotel, she treats everyone with a tender love and care (TLC) from the high rollers to the janitors and even the homeless people that the average person typically ignores, believing that everyone deserves to be treated humanely. She is always kind, and never has a bad day where she snaps at anyone, despite what she has going on in her personal life. Michelle's life is a testament to the extraordinary strength found within Black women. Every morning, Michelle navigates a maze of public transportation to reach her workplace, but not before making breakfast, packing lunches, helping with last minute homework, getting her children ready for school, and seeing them off. She works long hours to support her family, often dealing with microaggressions and biases that subtly permeate her daily interactions. She has been sexually *harassed and assaulted on many occasions throughout her 20-year tenure at this hotel. But as a single mother, she balances her job with the responsibilities of raising her children, ensuring they have a stable and loving home, and has no choice but to deal with it. She's been beaten, mugged, and left for dead on many a night on her way home and has still went to work the next morning. She goes to church on Sunday's, cooks meals for the homeless and everyone in the neighborhood, and everyone loves and respects her.*

~

Michelle's story is a poignant example of resilience in action. In a world where racial disparities persist, where the intersectionality of her identity as a black woman brings unique hurdles, she thrives despite the odds stacked against her. Her resilience is not just about persevering; it's about flourishing in the face of adversity. Her story is an inspiration to everyone in her community, but that's not why she does it. Her resilience is not a choice, it's a means of survival. Her paycheck when she works full-time, still often stretches thinner than she would like, which is why she has no choice but to work overtime any time it's offered. Being tired, taking breaks, self-care, are all not an option for her. If she doesn't work 60+ hours a week, there's bills that don't get paid. And even though she works so hard, she still had times when she's come home, and the lights were off or there was no hot water.

Through her determination and unwavering love for her family, Michelle's resilience shines brightly. She embodies the strength to confront challenges head-on, to challenge stereotypes, and to inspire those around her with her unwavering spirit. Her story resonates with countless Black women who, like her, rise above adversity with grace and courage. People call her "ma" and even though they all respect and look out for her, respect doesn't pay the bills.

As we delve into the importance of resilience for Black women, it is voices like Michelle's that remind us of the profound strength that resides within. It is their resilience, forged through the crucible of life's trials, that paves the way for progress and serves as a beacon of hope for generations.

Quick disclaimer: I am not stating that black women are more resilient than other races, I am simply a black woman so I can only speak to what I know. This book is not to offend anyone, resilience can be found within all women, but if you feel offended, this might not be the book for you.

Introduction to the resilience of a black woman

Amidst the tapestry of human experiences, there exists a group of individuals who have elevated resilience into an art form and deserve to be celebrated for their beauty and grace: Black women. Their journey through life is a testament to the remarkable strength that resides within them, a strength born not merely from choice but from necessity. The resilience of Black women, which runs deep in their veins, is both a survival mechanism and a learned behavior, shaped by the unique challenges they face in a society where the intersection of race, gender, and socioeconomic status casts long shadows.

Why must Black women be resilient? The answer is etched into the fabric of history and woven into the tapestry of their daily lives. Centuries of systemic inequalities, racial discrimination, and gender biases have carved a path laden with obstacles. From the echoes of slavery to the persistent struggles for civil rights, the historical burden borne by Black women has been profound. Their resilience is a response to this weight, a survival mechanism born from the need to navigate a world where opportunity and equality are not always freely given. There's always a catch to the freedom, for example, you can work outside of the home now, but because you're a black woman, you're going to get paid less than the average woman. You're going to be allowed in the same spaces, but you're not going to be allowed the same freedoms as another woman. Although not all black women are poor and struggling, the rich must start from somewhere, and you don't lose your resiliency just because you no longer need it. It is simply no longer a survival mechanism in the same way it is for other women. It can be used as a positive trait and even a compliment, instead of something that is necessary in daily life, and interchange between the ways in which they need to be resilient. Yet, they still are not as equal as a cisgendered male or white female counterparts.

Resilience for Black women is not just a trait; it is a way of life, a learned behavior passed down through generations. It is watching mothers, grandmothers, and sisters navigate the complexities of their existence with unwavering strength. It is witnessing these matriarchs face adversity head-on, forging pathways of survival and progress, and understanding that resilience is both a shield and a sword. Resilience acts as a shield, serving as a buffer against the emotional toll of challenges, helping Black women maintain their mental and emotional wellbeing even in the face of adversity. It shields them from the harm that discrimination and stereotypes can inflict, because these challenges were learned to be expected, and it enables them to maintain their sense of self and purpose. This does not at all mean that Black women are bulletproof, we are still emotional human beings, we are just taught to ignore the comments, racial slurs, and biases. We are forced to come from a place of understanding, that "they were just raised differently", "they're not used to seeing black people", or whatever sort of excuse we're taught to use to explain that person's behavior as acceptable, even when it's not. But after a while, even the strongest shield can eventually be dented and bended and not as functional as it used to be, which is where mental illness comes in.

However, resilience can also be used as a sword, which means that it becomes a tool for empowerment and progress. It equipes Black women with the strength and determination to confront obstacles head-on. Like a sword, resilience can be wielded to challenge stereotypes, break down barriers, and carve out pathways to success. It empowers Black women to be advocates for themselves and their communities, enabling them to fight for justice, equality, and the recognition of their worth. Resilience becomes a means of asserting agency, taking control of their own narratives, and driving change.

In this dual role, resilience becomes a dynamic force in the lives of Black women. It shields them from the harm of discrimination while simultaneously arming them with the strength to overcome adversity and drive positive change. It is both a form of self-preservation and a tool for empowerment, highlighting its multifaceted significance in the journey towards equality and wellbeing. Both the shield and the sword are necessary to fight the battles that the world throws at the Black woman. It is about the acknowledgement that societal expectations and stereotypes often thrust upon them demand a continuous demonstration of strength. This learned behavior is a response to the persistent pressure to appear eternally strong, even when vulnerability lies beneath the surface. It is the art of balancing the weight of others' expectations while maintaining their own sense of self.

In celebrating the resilience of Black women, we explore a journey marked by adversity, triumph, and the indomitable spirit that defines their lives. We honor not only their strength but the lessons they impart about resilience as a means of survival and a source of empowerment. Their stories remind us that within the crucible of life's trials, resilience is a beacon of hope, a testament to the human capacity to rise above and illuminate the path forward. Take a second to do the first journal prompt, before going through the personal stories of resilience of black women.

Journal Prompt #1

Reflect on a challenging moment in your life when you were forced to be resilient. What circumstances or obstacles did you face, and how did you navigate them? What did you learn about yourself during that experience, and how has it shaped your resilience today? Take time to journal your thoughts, emotions, and the lessons you can draw from your own journey to resilience.

Highlighting the unique strengths and qualities of Black women

"I don't have to check in on you because I knew you were okay. You're strong." A compliment right? No. Well at least not to me, and here's why. Just because I seem strong, doesn't mean that I am. But even if I am strong, that doesn't mean that I want to be. I actually don't. I am still a woman, one who values embodying the soft life. A vulnerable, emotional, heart-centered human being who goes through things. I am a single mother of a 1-year-old. I am a full-time therapist. I am a full-time graduate student. I am a full-time coach-in-training. I go through things, just as much as anyone else, and even though I "should know what to do because [I'm] a therapist", doesn't mean I always do. In fact, therapists are sometimes oblivous to their own personal and family traumas. We either over-diagnosis or think that nothing's wrong because we don't fit the textbook definition of a diagnosis.

The point is, I want, and even crave the support. And this is actually something that other black women experience from family and friends as well, the need for support, but the lack thereof. It goes back to the notion that black women are forced to be seen as resilient, and invincible, never needing help with anything.

I admit to needing help. I don't want to be a rough and tough strong independent woman all the time. I want the soft life, where I am taken care of and catered to, at least to some extent. Unleashing your inner light isn't about becoming selfish or becoming so full of yourself that you don't let people in. It's about learning to embrace the things that you are good at and enjoy doing, and letting go and delegating the things that you don't enjoy. Either way though, you are still not less of a woman.

You can be a great mom and still have someone else watch your kids every weekend for me time or for time alone with your partner. You can be a successful boss babe and still not wear all the hats in your business. It's about a balance, and learning to accept help, which I know, can sometimes be the hardest thing to do, but here's what happens when you don't delegate.

Understanding the Mental Health Crisis Among Women

As we've already mentioned before, we know that mental illness is an issue on the rise and typically ignored, but within mental illness and often a trigger or cause for a mental health disorder is a mental health crisis. "A mental health crisis is defined as an acute disruption of psychological homeostasis in which one's usual coping mechanisms fail, with evidence of distress and functional impairment. It is a person's subjective reaction to a stressful life experience that compromises their ability to cope or function" (Ernstmeyer and Christman, 2022).

There are 4 different crises that we can experience maturational, situational, adventitious, or sociocultural. In this book, I'm mainly going to focus on situational and maturational crises. "A situational crisis (also referred to as an accidental or external crisis) results from unanticipated, sudden, or unavoidable events that largely affect a person's identity and roles, and revolves around grief, usually from a loss of an established situation that threatens a person physically, socially, or psychologically" (Ernstmeyer and Christman, 2022). This can include divorce, unexpected job loss, change in financial status, academic failure, mental illness, birth of a child with a disability or other healthcare issues, death of a child or family members, serious injury, or diagnosis of a chronic or terminal illness.

In 2023, I had a lot of these going on at once: a mental illness, a birth of my son prematurely which resulted in multiple health issues, and I experienced a change in financial status. These issues also relate to situational crises in young adulthood which include:

- Leaving home
- Continuing one's education.
- Getting started in an occupation.
- Marriage
- Managing a home
- Pregnancy
- Childbirth

Again, I check off the boxes of continuing my education by going back for another master's, getting started in my occupation because I started a position as a therapist at a new agency, I was pregnant and then experienced a traumatic childbirth, and we went through an eviction while my son was in the NICU so I had to hurriedly get my first apartment in my name and pay all the bills on my own, providing for me, my mom, and my son for the first time which is managing a home. Naturally, all the stress resulted in my previous struggle with mental health, specifically depression coming to a head. But I also experienced severe anxiety for the first time and at one point I had 3 panic attacks in less than a month, one while at work.

That was when I knew I could no longer suffer in silence, it was my body's cry for help. As Bessel van der Kolk mentioned in a training course I did with him in December of 2023 and he even has a book on it titled "The Body Keeps the Score", and mine was struggling to keep up with all of life's changes. So, I sought out a therapist that the NICU was offering to parents whose children had an extended stay and although I had a terrible experience with said therapist, I did receive clarity on my mental status.

Here is a quote from the therapist's text message, word for word as she had written it "Your assessment results indicate that you are experiencing severe depression as well as severe anxiety." This single sentence was a life-altering revelation for me at the time. Instead of being alarming, it brought me so much peace and solace because I finally could put a name to the symptoms I was experiencing.

For those of you who are unfamiliar with depression and anxiety, both are on a spectrum, meaning that there are varying types of depression and anxiety, as well as variations in severity level. Depending on which test you are given for Major Depressive Disorder (MDD), there are usually always at least 3 levels of depression that they will be scoring for: mild (which is 5 symptoms and the minimum criteria to receive the diagnosis), moderate (6 to 7 symptoms), and severe (8 to 9 symptoms), but there are different questions used on each test. The particular test that I was administered for MDD included an extreme level which I was 1 point away from scoring. I do want to admit that assessment occurred 2 to 3 months after my mental health had initially started to deteriorate, so in hindsight I knew I had probably had the highest score for depression and anxiety possible. As a therapist and really even a layman who is educated about mental health and what certain disorders look like, tell you never to self-diagnose, always go get a professional's opinion, so even though I knew what I had been struggling with, I wasn't allowed to fully make that distinction. However, what I did do was, recognizing that I was struggling, I decided to be proactive in self-healing through journaling, reaching out to my support system, and a lot of the tools I am going to teach you here.

The crazy part was, later in the year in about August or September, a female client requested to change therapists reporting that "I don't know what changed but ever since she had her baby, she seems a little off." Hmm, I wonder why...Let's unpack it.

I started my job while in final trimesters of pregnancy. They knew I would be having a baby and need time off which is why I took the job in the first place. However, I was not prepared for my birthing experience, though I know none of us ever really are. My water broke prematurely and I thought I peed on myself and just couldn't stop peeing, and still going to work for a week or two straight. Eventually, I had painful distractions which started on a Saturday and drastically increased by Sunday afternoon, and me fearfully admitting to my mom that I was worried and rushing to the Emergency Room. We thought it would simply be an overnight or few day stay, but yet as soon as they triaged me, I ended up being admitted. We found out at some point that it was a premature rupture and since I was only 27 weeks, it was way too soon to have my baby so we agreed that I would stay in the hospital for 6-8 weeks till I was at least 36-38 weeks. Mind you I had just gotten my job and hadn't even been there a month which is why I was even reluctant to go to the ER in the first place. I had been contemplating it and silently fighting the pain since Saturday to fear that they would fire me (again another situational crisis), so I got permission from my amazing boss and HR to work from the hospital for the next few weeks until I had my baby.

Less than a week in, things took a turn for the worse and my baby wasn't breathing properly, so they scheduled me for an emergency C-section. The night that he turned 28-weeks, as soon as it hit midnight, I was rushed into surgery. Another trauma. Oh, but I skipped the part where when I first got admitted and the OB's were trying to check how dilated I was, and painfully and against my will, forced multiple fingers into my already swollen vagina and had me literally screaming and fighting for my life while I was pinned down like a mental patient for the procedure for 2-5 minutes, going against their promise not to hurt me and force anything on to me. And though not a big deal to some, I had never felt so disempowered.

That was probably the biggest and most traumatic trauma, which we call a capital 't' trauma. That was all pre-birth, though, it got much, much worse after my baby actually came which we'll talk more about later but going back to the previous point. Having experienced all this, I wonder why I changed? I was 24, had never been admitted to the hospital or had any serious health problems EVER, and there were multiple times I was told everything was okay by medical staff and then it wasn't, and I know there's plenty of other women out there who've experienced mistrust from the healthcare professionals as well.

Mind you, I had just gotten used to the fact that I was going to working from a hospital for the next 8 weeks. On top of that, I had just started my job and hadn't been there even a month yet, so I thought for sure I was going to be a new mother and be homeless.

There was just so much on my mind, I was scared, I felt overwhelmed, I was upset because I felt that the doctors didn't know what was going on (which was true because everyday they were telling me something different). On top of that, a neonatologist had just come by that day and told me the ultrasounds were looking good and that the baby was okay. There was just so much back and forth that my physical and mental health were definitely out of wack.

Fast forward, the C-section goes well, I have the baby and he's not breathing on his own. I just had my firstborn and I was so traumatized and scared he wouldn't make it, and I didn't even get to see him when that was probably the most important thing to me at that time. As a matter of fact, it wasn't until about 2 or 3 months later, closer to the end of his hospital stay when I first held him. Imagine being a new mom and having your son in the hospital for 99 days and you can only hold his little finger through an incubator and change his diapers every 3 hours (depending on the nurse).

Well that was the extent of motherhood for my son's first 3 months of his life until June 1st when he finally got out of the hospital. Mind you, I only took off for a few days, maybe a week max after having him, and proceeded to work from the hospital afterwards because it was a new job and I couldn't afford to get fired. And even once I was discharged, I stayed in my son's hospital room for the first month of his life, only going home for like a day before going back.

I say all this to say that she was right, I was not okay at all after having him. I WAS GOING THROUGH IT and I knew that, but to say something 6 months later after I was trying to get into the routine of being a new mom and still keep my first real full-time job. I was trying my damnedest to be okay and to do everything expected of me, and to not let things get to me, but I was messed up. To anyone who has never had a firstborn preemie, you just have to imagine that it was hard. I can't even explain how I was feeling, but I don't wish this on any mother, and I know that my situation wasn't as bad as some other mothers, but it was bad for me. It was terrible for me. I was 25, still living with my mom, and not at all prepared for any of it. I did the best that I could and it just sucked that some people didn't appreciate it. But that's okay. Not everyone is going to acknowledge you.

I was severely depressed and having panic attacks in between breaks at work. I was (breast)pumping at work and going through postpartum something, I don't even know what, but it was definitely postpartum mental health struggles. I was somehow functioning on autopilot though not mentally functional. My point is that often times we are suffering in silence and those around us don't even know or can't gage how bad it is, so it's up for us to learn how to articulate that to them or to ask for help.

Having these 2 diagnoses gave me peace because I told myself "At least I'm not crazy. At least I'm not imagining these symptoms, this is really as bad as I thought it was." Because that was another thing too, I cried out for help, multiple times to loved ones, medical staff, anyone, and everyone, long before I did therapy and stressed to them that I wasn't okay and that I couldn't cope with it all. At one point I even had suicidal thoughts and ideations, and every single person I told downplayed it and told me I'd get through it. My story isn't just a tale about the medical system, it's about a struggle and lack of support from my entire world at that time. I truly went through these struggles and came out on the other end, by myself.

I decided that I didn't want to do therapy anymore because I was qualified to deal with everything by myself, and I honestly probably should have done therapy. But I coached myself back to being okay again, and then after being okay, I coached myself into becoming happy and being at peace. And even though I'm not happy 24/7 and still have bouts of depression every once in a while, there's no more panic attacks and I am at peace.

I'm at peace with myself for everything that led me to this point, the things I could control and even those that I couldn't. I'm at peace with the doctors and nurses at that hospital who drove me crazy at times, and especially with those who gave me unwavering support when I really needed it. I'm at peace with my son's absent father. I'm just peaceful. And I know now that everything that happened had to happen in order to make me the woman that I am today.

My hopes are that you walk away from this chapter with the beginning stages of peace and forgiveness for yourself and everything that you have had to endure. I'm not saying it'll be easy, but it is a necessary part of the journey. Take as much time as you need, journal, write a letter, cry, let out the anger, do whatever you need to do. And day-by-day, it'll get easier.

Sidenote

I just want to take a second to say that when my water broke, I said to myself "What if my water just broke" and my mom had made a joke about it, but again with this being my first pregnancy, I didn't know what to expect, and it was definitely not like the movies. Then a week or two before my water broke, I had gone to get an ultrasound for a routine prenatal checkup and my ultrasound tech was concerned then because my son had started to kick and was already trying to break the sac. But instead of sending me home with any precautions or extra measures, they just left me and my eager-to-be-out-of-the-womb baby to our own devices. There was so much oversight that occurred throughout my pregnancy, and I take fault for my part in it all because I was definitely worried and should have spoken up sooner. I admit that, definitely learned my lesson, 1,000x over. Ladies, if you feel like something is wrong, like I said before, trust your intuition, always seek help, and don't just blindly ignore it. Too often, mental health providers shine off our suspicions, but please always get a second opinion or a tenth, don't stop until your concerns are addressed. It's okay to not know something, it's okay to reach out for help. Please do, I'm begging you to.

The importance of mental health awareness

Mental health awareness, particularly among women, is of paramount importance for several compelling reasons which we've all pretty much discussed. So here's what mental health awareness looks like:

- Education and Information Sharing: Mental health awareness involves disseminating accurate information about mental health conditions, symptoms, and available resources. This can be done through workshops, seminars, educational materials, and online resources, aiming to increase understanding and reduce stigma surrounding mental health issues.

- Promotion of Self-Care Practices: Encouraging individuals to prioritize self-care practices that nurture mental well-being is an essential aspect of mental health awareness. This includes activities such as exercise, mindfulness, journaling, spending time in nature, and maintaining healthy boundaries in relationships.

- Open Dialogue and Communication: Creating spaces for open dialogue about mental health allows individuals to share their experiences, struggles, and triumphs without fear of judgment or stigma. This can occur in various settings, including support groups, community events, social media platforms, and workplace wellness programs.

- Advocacy and Activism: Mental health awareness involves advocating for policy changes and initiatives that promote mental health equity, access to care, and destigmatization. This can include lobbying for increased funding for mental health services, supporting legislation that protects the rights of individuals with mental health conditions, and challenging discriminatory practices.

- Cultural Sensitivity and Inclusivity: Recognizing the diverse cultural backgrounds and experiences of individuals is crucial in mental health awareness efforts. This involves promoting culturally sensitive approaches to mental health care, providing services in multiple languages, and addressing systemic barriers that disproportionately affect marginalized communities.

- Media Representation and Campaigns: Media campaigns, documentaries, and storytelling play a significant role in raising awareness about mental health issues and challenging stereotypes. By portraying diverse and authentic representations of mental health experiences, media can help reduce stigma and increase empathy and understanding.

- Training and Professional Development: Providing training and resources for mental health professionals, educators, employers, and first responders equips them with the knowledge and skills to support individuals experiencing mental health challenges effectively. This can include training in trauma-informed care, suicide prevention, and recognizing signs of distress.

- Integration into Various Settings: Incorporating mental health awareness into various settings, such as schools, workplaces, healthcare settings, and community organizations, ensures that individuals have access to information and support where they spend their time.

As we know, children spend a lot of their time at home in their early years, and look to their parents for guidance. So how do we talk about mental health in the home?

- Normalize the Conversation: Start by normalizing discussions about mental health within your family. Emphasize that it's okay to talk about emotions, struggles, and challenges, and that seeking help for mental health concerns is a sign of strength, not weakness.

- Create a Safe and Supportive Environment: Choose a time and place where everyone feels comfortable and relaxed. Encourage open communication by listening attentively, validating feelings, and expressing empathy and understanding.

- Use Age-Appropriate Language: Tailor your language and explanations to the age and developmental level of your children. Use simple and concrete language for younger children, while providing more detailed information for older children and teenagers.

- Honest and Authentic: Be honest and authentic when discussing mental health with your children and loved ones. Share your own experiences and emotions in an age-appropriate manner, emphasizing that it's normal to experience a range of feelings and that everyone needs support sometimes.

- Provide Education and Information: Offer age-appropriate information about mental health conditions, symptoms, and available resources. Use books, videos, and online resources geared towards children and teenagers to help explain complex concepts in an accessible way. I will soon be coming out with children's books specifically made for mental health. Follow me on @_theradianteffect on Instagram to stay in tune. I will also provide worksheets and scripts to help start the conversation.

- Encourage Questions and Discussion: Encourage your children and loved ones to ask questions and share their thoughts and feelings about mental health. Foster a non-judgmental atmosphere where everyone feels comfortable expressing themselves and seeking clarification.

- Model Healthy Coping Strategies: Lead by example by modeling healthy coping strategies and self-care practices. Show your children and loved ones how to manage stress, regulate emotions, and seek support when needed.

- Address Stigma and Misconceptions: Challenge stigma and misconceptions about mental health by providing accurate information, correcting stereotypes, and emphasizing the importance of empathy, compassion, and acceptance.

- Seek Professional Help When Needed: If you or a family member is struggling with mental health issues, don't hesitate to seek professional help. Reach out to a therapist, counselor, or mental health provider who can offer support and guidance tailored to your family's needs.

The prevalence of mental health challenges among women

"Women are also twice as likely as men to be diagnosed with panic disorder (PD), which affects 6 million U.S. adults, and with specific phobias, which impact 19 million adults in the U.S. The prevalence of serious mental illness is almost 70% greater in women than in men" (Regis College Online) . In fact, the National Institute of Mental Health states that certain mental health disorders "such as depression, anxiety, and eating disorders" are more common in women. A study done in 2021 showed that there is approximately a minimum of 9.6% and maximum of 69.3% of women with common mental health disorders. (Bezerra, Héllyda de Souza et al. "Prevalence and Associated Factors of Common Mental Disorders in Women: A Systematic Review." Public health reviews vol. 42 1604234. 23 Aug. 2021, doi:10.3389/phrs.2021.1604234). "The studies included in this review showed multiple factors associated with CMD, however, only a few stood out, namely, unemployment, low income, low education level, smoking, marital status, experiences of violence, and poor self-rated health. These findings were explained by the different social, economic, demographic conditions and access to health services in the countries (2021)."

Biologically, hormonal fluctuations throughout the menstrual cycle, pregnancy, childbirth, and menopause can significantly impact women's mental well-being. For example, postpartum depression affects approximately 10-15% of women after giving birth, highlighting the unique challenges faced during the perinatal period. Additionally, women are more susceptible to certain autoimmune disorders, which are often linked to increased rates of depression and anxiety.

Psychologically, societal expectations and gender norms can contribute to women's vulnerability to mental health struggles. Pressures related to caregiving, career advancement, body image, and relationship dynamics can create stressors that predispose women to conditions such as generalized anxiety disorder and eating disorders. Moreover, societal stigma surrounding mental health may discourage women from seeking help, leading to underdiagnosis and undertreatment of their conditions.

Socio-cultural factors also play a significant role in women's mental health. Discrimination, gender-based violence, socioeconomic disparities, and lack of access to healthcare can exacerbate stressors and increase the risk of mental health disorders among women, particularly those from marginalized communities.

Furthermore, intersectionality must be considered when examining mental health disparities among women. Women of color, LGBTQ+ women, women with disabilities, and other marginalized groups often face compounded challenges that can further impact their mental well-being.

Culturally, women often face unique barriers that can make it challenging to seek help from mental health professionals. These barriers are deeply rooted in societal norms, cultural expectations, and gender roles, which can vary significantly across different communities and cultures. One prominent barrier is the stigma surrounding mental health within many cultures. Mental health issues are sometimes viewed as a taboo topic, associated with weakness, shame, or moral failing. As a result, women may fear judgment or discrimination if they openly acknowledge their struggles or seek professional help.

This stigma can be particularly widely accepted in cultures where mental health is not widely understood or accepted, leading to silence and secrecy around mental health issues. For example, in the black communities, mental health is something that isn't really talked about on a regular basis, especially with youth. If depression or anxiety is brought up by a teacher or other school professional, the parent might say "Oh, they were just playing or being dramatic." It might not be properly addressed or taken seriously. It wasn't even until I was an adult when I saw my mom openly talking about and going to therapy, after I was already in school for it.

Additionally, traditional gender roles often dictate that women prioritize the well-being of others over their own. Women are frequently expected to fulfill caregiving roles and maintain harmony within the family, which can leave little time or energy for addressing their own mental health needs. Seeking help for mental health concerns may be perceived as a selfish act or a sign of failure to meet societal expectations, further discouraging women from reaching out for support.

Furthermore, cultural factors such as language barriers, lack of culturally competent mental health services, and limited access to resources can also hinder women's ability to seek help. Women from immigrant or minority communities may face additional challenges in finding mental health professionals who understand their cultural background, beliefs, and values, making it difficult to feel understood and supported in therapy.

Addressing the prevalence of mental health struggles among women requires a comprehensive approach that addresses biological, psychological, and socio-cultural factors. This includes promoting gender-sensitive healthcare services, increasing access to mental health resources, challenging societal norms that contribute to stigma, and advocating for policies that support women's mental well-being across diverse populations.

Additionally, raising awareness and fostering open discussions about women's mental health can help reduce stigma and encourage early intervention and support. Creating safe spaces for open dialogue about mental health within communities and challenging stigma through education and advocacy can also help empower women to seek the support they need without fear or shame. Ultimately, breaking down these cultural barriers requires a collaborative effort involving mental health professionals, community leaders, policymakers, and individuals themselves to promote acceptance, understanding, and support for women's mental health.

My hopes are that this book can be the first steps in opening that dialogue and creating safe spaces for families to talk about mental health. The journals and products that are made as companions for this book, as well as the courses and eBooks that will come after it, will teach not only you, but your family members how to communicate more effectively.

The truth is that therapy is not for everybody, and therapy isn't actually what a lot of people choose to turn to as a first resort, but that doesn't mean that the work isn't important. And people will come to therapy, when they are ready. A lot of people try to fix themselves through YouTube videos, shadow work/inner child healing, and journaling. These are all great ways to get started with your mental health repairment. What's the difference between a therapist and a coach?

Do I need a therapist or a coach?

Therapists and coaches both work with individuals to support personal growth, development, and well-being, but there are distinct differences in their roles, approaches, and qualifications.

Therapists typically focus on addressing mental health issues, emotional challenges, and psychological disorders. They often work with clients to explore past experiences, identify underlying issues, and develop coping strategies to manage symptoms. Therapists may use various therapeutic modalities, such as cognitive-behavioral therapy (CBT), psychodynamic therapy, or mindfulness-based approaches, depending on the needs of the client.

In contrast, coaches primarily focus on helping clients set and achieve specific goals, whether personal or professional. Coaches often work in areas such as career development, leadership skills, relationship building, time management, and overall life satisfaction. While coaches may address some emotional issues that arise in the pursuit of goals, they typically do not delve into deep-seated psychological issues or provide treatment for mental health disorders. Actually, we are typically told not to.

Therapists typically hold advanced degrees in psychology, counseling, social work, or related fields. They undergo extensive training, including graduate education, supervised clinical experience, and licensure or certification requirements, depending on their jurisdiction. Therapists are trained to assess, diagnose, and treat mental health conditions using evidence-based therapeutic techniques.

On the other hand, coaches come from diverse backgrounds and may have varying levels of formal training and education. While some coaches hold certifications from coaching programs or professional organizations, coaching is currently an unregulated field, meaning there are no standardized licensure or educational requirements. However, reputable coaching programs often provide comprehensive training in coaching methodologies, ethics, and practical skills. I, personally, choose to have my certifications in coaching, and am already certified as a Master Transformation Coach and Master Mindfulness Coach, while working on getting my ICF credentials. I specialize in mindset and transformation (if not already clear), but also with a faith-based perspective.

The client relationship in therapy is typically characterized by a professional, therapeutic alliance focused on healing and personal growth. Therapists maintain strict confidentiality and adhere to ethical guidelines to create a safe and supportive environment for clients to explore their thoughts, feelings, and experiences. In contrast, coaches typically work in a collaborative partnership with clients, providing guidance, support, and accountability as clients work towards their goals. While the relationship may be supportive, it is generally less structured than the therapeutic relationship, and coaches may incorporate more direct feedback and action-oriented strategies to facilitate progress.

In summary, while therapists and coaches both play valuable roles in supporting individuals in their personal development and well-being, their approaches, training, and focus areas differ significantly. Therapists primarily address mental health issues and emotional challenges using evidence-based therapeutic techniques, while coaches focus on goal-setting, skill-building, and achievement in various areas of life.

You can always have both a therapist and a coach, but typically if you are emotionally unstable and struggling with any serious mental illness, especially severe depression and suicidal ideation, you must go to a therapist. Whereas, if you are simply struggling with happiness and fulfillment, but generally don't have any sort of mental breakdowns, a coach might be more beneficial for you. Therapists do, however, work with an array of mental health struggles (whether mild or severe), so when in doubt, always try a therapist first.

A lot of the ways in which I coach and practice therapy are similar, in that, I am wanting to help the client develop resilience and inner strength and confidence to deal with their struggles on their own. The goal with all my clients, is to build resilience from within, and never need me again.

Find what works best for you in that season, but don't be afraid to try new things.

Chapter 2: Cultivating Resilience from Within

As women, we often find ourselves navigating a myriad of challenges, from societal expectations to personal struggles, that test our resilience and inner strength. Cultivating resilience from within is not merely a survival mechanism; it is a transformative journey of self-discovery, empowerment, and growth. In this chapter, we delve into the unique experiences and perspectives of women on their path to resilience, exploring the ways in which they harness their inner resources to overcome adversity and thrive in the face of challenges.

Yet, we are all no strangers to adversity. We face societal pressures, gender biases, and cultural expectations that shape our experiences and perceptions of ourselves. Within each of us lies a wellspring of resilience – a deep reservoir of strength, courage, and perseverance that enables us to rise above adversity and emerge stronger than before.

At the heart of cultivating resilience from within is the journey of self-discovery and self-empowerment. It is about uncovering our innate resilience, tapping into our inner wisdom, and embracing our unique strengths and capabilities. Through introspection, reflection, and self-care practices, we learn to nurture and cultivate our resilience, building a solid foundation that sustains us through life's storms.

We will share stories of triumph and resilience throughout this chapter, highlighting the resilience of women from diverse backgrounds and walks of life. Through these narratives, we hope to inspire and empower women to acknowledge the ways in which you are already resilient in everyday life, and then hone in on those skills in the areas you feel weakest in.

Remember this book is not about reinventing the wheel or creating something new inside you, it is about unleashing what is already engrained in you.

Resilience is the key to overcoming adversity

Resilience is not just a trait; it's a vital part of our inner strength, enabling us to navigate the turbulent waters of life. It is the ability to bounce back from setbacks, adapt to challenges, and emerge stronger and wiser from experiences of adversity. This chapter explores the essence of resilience and provides practical strategies to cultivate it, empowering you to face life's difficulties with unwavering strength and grace.

Understanding Resilience

Resilience is often misunderstood as simply being tough or unyielding. However, true resilience is about flexibility, adaptability, and growth. It's not about avoiding stress or hardship, because these things are inevitable, but rather about learning how to manage and thrive despite them. The goal is to be able to not let stress stunt your growth, and make you feel stuck, we'd rather you accept hardship as part of the process (a growing pain if you will), something you expected and created a plan to move around. But honestly, you're probably already doing it. That it is to say, you're probably already practicing resilience on a day-to-day basis without acknowledging it as such, and it's simply a norm to you.

Typically, we are all resilient in some way, shape, or form for simply having made it to the point in which we are in life, such as:

1. Balancing Multiple Roles

Every day, women manage the complexities of being employees, caregivers, friends, and individuals with personal dreams and goals. Resilience is shown in how we adapt to shifting priorities, find creative solutions, and keep moving forward even when the demands feel overwhelming and it seems like we have no way out. Balancing multiple roles requires a constant recalibration of energy and focus, which demonstrates immense inner strength and perseverance. It's not easy to balance multiple roles, especially as a mother, but somehow we still do it.

2. Advocating for Ourselves and Others

Speaking up, whether for ourselves or someone else, often requires courage in environments that may not always be supportive. Resilience is in the ability to assert our needs, challenge injustices, and claim space despite fear of rejection or criticism. Each time we advocate, we prove our strength in pushing boundaries and fighting for what we feel is right, and ultimately, what we deserve.

3. Managing Emotional Labor

Women often take on the unspoken responsibility of maintaining emotional harmony in relationships, offering comfort, and anticipating the needs of others. This ongoing effort, though invisible, requires emotional resilience and the capacity to prioritize others even when our own energy is low. It reflects a strength rooted in empathy and care, despite it being physically and emotionally taxing.

4. Persisting Through Everyday Challenges

Whether it's navigating subtle microaggressions at work or overcoming societal barriers, women encounter obstacles that test their resolve daily. Resilience is shown in how we persevere—choosing not to give up, seeking solutions, and finding ways to thrive in environments that may not always be fair or inclusive.

- *Breaking Through Workplace Inequalities*

Women often face wage gaps, underrepresentation in leadership roles, and biases that undervalue their contributions. Resilience is shown when women pursue higher education, advocate for promotions, negotiate salaries, or step into male-dominated fields despite these systemic challenges.

- *Defying Gender Stereotypes*

Society often imposes rigid expectations about how women should behave, dress, or live. Women overcome these barriers by embracing their individuality—whether it's choosing a career over traditional roles, pursuing unconventional hobbies, or speaking out against judgment. Each act of defiance is a testament to inner strength and authenticity.

- *Challenging Beauty Standards*

Women are constantly bombarded with unrealistic ideals of beauty, which can harm self-esteem. Resilience is seen in women who reject these standards by embracing their natural selves, advocating for body positivity, and building self-worth based on their character, not their appearance.

• *Navigating Cultural Expectations*
In some cultures, women may face restrictions on education, career choices, or personal freedoms. Those who pursue their dreams despite these limitations—whether by attending school, starting a business, or choosing their own path in life —demonstrate immense bravery and perseverance.
• *Advocating for Reproductive Rights*
Women around the world face challenges accessing reproductive healthcare or making decisions about their own bodies. Resilience is reflected in how they advocate for their rights, educate themselves and others, and support organizations that fight for change, even in hostile environments.
• *Fighting for Representation*
Women often work tirelessly to amplify their voices and ensure representation in politics, media, and other influential spaces. Whether running for office, producing content that reflects authentic female perspectives, or supporting movements like #MeToo, they actively dismantle systems of exclusion.
• *Balancing Motherhood and Ambition*
Society often pressures women to prioritize family over career, or vice versa, creating impossible standards. Resilience is evident in women who refuse to choose— managing both roles with grace, advocating for parental leave policies, and proving that success doesn't require sacrificing one for the other.

5. Showing Up Despite Exhaustion

Caring for a sick child, meeting deadlines at work, or supporting a loved one while feeling mentally or physically drained highlights a unique strength. Resilience here is about enduring difficult moments with grace, even when it feels like there's little energy left to give. It's a testament to our dedication and love for those we care about.

6. Overcoming Self-Doubt

Self-doubt can often whisper that we're not good enough, yet women consistently push past these fears to achieve their goals. Resilience is in silencing that inner critic, trying again after failures, and continuing to believe in our potential, even when external validation feels scarce.

7. Creating Joy Amid Adversity

During challenging times, finding joy might seem impossible, yet women often create moments of beauty and celebration in their lives. Whether it's a small gesture like lighting a candle or hosting a family dinner, this resilience lies in the ability to find hope and positivity despite hardships. It's about refusing to let difficulties define our experience of life.

8. Adapting to Change

Life's transitions—becoming a mother, starting over after a breakup, or pursuing a new career—can feel destabilizing. Yet, resilience is shown in how women adjust to these changes, embrace uncertainty, and use the experience as a catalyst for growth. Each adaptation reflects our ability to rebuild and reimagine ourselves.

9. Supporting and Lifting Others

Even when we are carrying our own struggles, women often prioritize uplifting others—offering advice, mentorship, or a listening ear. This resilience stems from a deep sense of community and a belief in collective strength. By helping others rise, we demonstrate our ability to lead with compassion and perseverance.

The Distinct Forms of Resilience: Advocacy, Emotional Labor, and Empowerment

Advocating for others, managing emotional labor, and supporting and lifting others are interconnected but distinct ways in which women demonstrate resilience in their relationships and communities. Each reflects a unique aspect of emotional strength, highlighting different approaches to care and empowerment.

Advocating for others involves actively standing up for someone's rights, needs, or well-being in situations where they might lack the power to do so themselves. This could mean defending a colleague facing discrimination, speaking out against injustice, or using your voice to demand fairness in spaces where inequality persists. Advocacy is often outwardly visible and action-oriented, requiring courage and a willingness to confront uncomfortable or adversarial situations. It's about being a voice for change and showing resilience by standing firm in the face of resistance or societal pressures.

Managing emotional labor, on the other hand, is a quieter, less visible form of resilience. Emotional labor encompasses the ongoing effort to maintain harmony and emotional balance in relationships. This might involve checking in on loved ones, resolving conflicts, remembering special dates, or providing emotional support during difficult times. Unlike advocacy, which is direct and situational, emotional labor often happens in the background and requires constant emotional awareness and empathy. The resilience here lies in the ability to prioritize others' emotional well-being while managing your own, even when the work is invisible and underappreciated.

Supporting and lifting others focuses on empowerment and growth. This involves mentoring, sharing resources, encouraging someone to pursue their dreams, or celebrating their successes. While advocacy is about stepping in to protect or fight for someone, supporting others is about creating a space for them to advocate for themselves. It is more collaborative and celebratory, rooted in the belief that everyone deserves to thrive. Resilience in this context comes from fostering confidence in others, even while navigating your own challenges.

In essence, advocating for others is bold and systemic, emotional labor is empathetic and relational, and supporting others is empowering and future-focused. Together, these actions showcase the multifaceted ways women contribute to their relationships and communities, each requiring its own form of strength and determination.

The Role of Resilience in Overcoming Adversity

Adversity is an inevitable part of life. It can come in many forms, from personal loss and financial struggles to health issues and relationship problems. As we've discussed, resilience doesn't eliminate these challenges; instead, it changes how we respond to them. With resilience, we can:

• Maintain Perspective: Resilience helps us keep a balanced view, preventing us from becoming overwhelmed by the immediate pain or difficulty. It allows us to step back, evaluate the situation objectively, and avoid getting consumed by emotions.

• Stay Positive: It encourages a positive outlook, even in the darkest of times, helping us to see the potential for positive outcomes and learn from every experience. Resilience helps us understand that setbacks are often opportunities for growth and transformation.

• Adapt and Innovate: Resilience fosters adaptability, allowing us to adjust our plans and strategies in response to new realities. Whether it's modifying our goals or finding alternative solutions, resilience enables us to pivot without losing sight of our long-term vision.

• Build Strength: Every time we overcome a challenge, we build inner strength and confidence, making us better prepared for future adversities. The more we persevere, the more we realize our capabilities, strengthening our belief in ourselves.

• Develop Emotional Agility: Resilience helps us develop emotional agility, which is the ability to acknowledge and process our emotions without letting them control us. This emotional flexibility allows us to respond to difficult situations calmly, rather than reacting impulsively or getting stuck in negativity.

• Cultivate Patience: Through resilience, we learn to trust the process and understand that not all challenges can be resolved immediately. It teaches us to have patience with ourselves and the situation, recognizing that healing and growth take time.

• Foster a Growth Mindset: Resilience encourages us to adopt a growth mindset, where we see challenges as opportunities to learn and evolve. Rather than viewing adversity as something to avoid, we come to understand that it is a natural part of progress and personal development.

• Strengthen Relationships: As we face adversity, resilience also helps us strengthen our relationships by learning how to communicate more effectively, be supportive, and navigate conflicts with empathy and understanding. We lean on others and allow them to lean on us, creating deeper connections in the process.

These aspects of resilience not only help us navigate life's difficulties but also shape us into stronger, more capable individuals who can face challenges with grace and wisdom.

Building Resilience: Practical Strategies

Cultivating a growth mindset is fundamental to building resilience. This involves embracing challenges as opportunities to learn and grow, rather than as threats to our self-esteem. By viewing failures as stepping stones to success, we can shift our perspective from one of defeat to one of continuous improvement. Celebrating small victories along the way reinforces this mindset, acknowledging that progress is made in incremental steps, not giant leaps.

Developing strong relationships is another key component of resilience. Surrounding ourselves with supportive and positive people provides a network of encouragement and strength. It's important to remember that seeking help and leaning on others does not signify weakness; rather, it's a crucial part of resilience. Building reciprocal relationships, where support is both given and received, creates a robust support system that can help us navigate difficult times.

Practicing self-care is essential for maintaining resilience. Prioritizing physical health through regular exercise, a balanced diet, and sufficient rest lays a strong foundation for overall well-being. Equally important is engaging in activities that promote mental health, such as meditation, journaling, or pursuing hobbies that bring joy and relaxation. Setting boundaries to protect our time and energy ensures that we don't become overwhelmed by external demands.

Enhancing emotional awareness helps us build resilience by enabling us to understand and manage our emotions effectively. Developing a deep understanding of our emotional responses and their impact on our thoughts and behaviors allows us to stay grounded. Practicing mindfulness can help us remain present and reduce anxiety about the future or regrets about the past. Allowing ourselves to feel and process emotions, rather than suppressing them, is a crucial aspect of resilience, as it involves working through pain rather than avoiding it.

Setting realistic goals helps to build resilience by providing a clear and achievable path forward. Breaking down larger challenges into manageable tasks and setting achievable goals can prevent us from feeling overwhelmed. Celebrating even small achievements maintains motivation and a sense of progress. Remaining flexible and adjusting goals as needed is also important, as the path to success is rarely linear and often requires adaptability.

Finding meaning and purpose in our lives strengthens our resilience by giving us a sense of direction and motivation. Reflecting on our values and what truly matters to us can guide our actions and decisions. Engaging in activities and pursuits that align with our sense of purpose provides fulfillment and sustains us through difficult times. In moments of hardship, reminding ourselves of our larger goals and the bigger picture can help us stay focused and resilient.

Real Stories of Resilience

To truly understand the power of resilience, let's explore some real-life stories of individuals who have overcome significant adversity through sheer determination and resilience:

1. Maya Angelou: Despite facing racism, sexual abuse, and poverty, Maya Angelou became one of the most revered poets and authors in history. Her resilience allowed her to transform her pain into powerful words that continue to inspire millions.
2. Oprah Winfrey: Growing up in poverty and experiencing numerous hardships, Oprah Winfrey rose to become a media mogul and philanthropist. Her story exemplifies how resilience can lead to incredible success and impact.
3. Malala Yousafzai: After surviving a targeted attack by the Taliban, Malala Yousafzai continued her advocacy for girls' education with even greater fervor. Her resilience has made her a global symbol of courage and determination.

Though these women may seem like anomalies, resilience is within each and every one of us. To illustrate this point, I went through my family tree, conducting interviews to see what women in my family went through, and how they were resilient in everyday life. The places where I've bolder, usually in parentheses is where I've added to their though to clarify it/add my two cents.

Personal Story #1

Introducing Grandma again, sorry, not sorry y'all. In my teenage years and especially in young adulthood, my grandma was my favorite person. She was literally my rock, through a lot of the mental health struggles I experienced in high school, but in this chapter, we are going to see her in a different light. She taught me what it truly meant to be resilient, but here's what it was like for her to develop it:

Grandma didn't just wake up one day being the strong, unwavering woman I came to know and admire. Her resilience wasn't something she was born with—it was something she had to cultivate over the years through her own trials and tribulations. From raising children on her own, managing financial hardships, to facing personal losses, she learned early on that life wasn't going to hand her anything easy. And yet, she never once complained. She didn't have the luxury of dwelling in her pain or frustration. Instead, she turned those experiences into lessons, using each hardship as an opportunity to grow stronger.

Her resilience was shaped by countless moments of struggle, but it was also nurtured by her faith, her ability to adapt, and her deep sense of responsibility to her family. She taught me that resilience doesn't mean never break down—it means knowing how to pick yourself up, adjust, and keep moving forward, no matter the obstacle. There were times when I saw her go through things that most people would crumble under, yet she carried on, never letting her circumstances define her.

What stood out most about Grandma's resilience was her mindset. She didn't view her challenges as roadblocks; she viewed them as stepping stones to something greater. And through it all, she never lost sight of the importance of community—whether it was leaning on her friends, family, or simply showing up for others, Grandma understood that resilience is not just about individual strength, but about leaning on those around you. She was the epitome of quiet strength, teaching me that true resilience lies in the ability to endure, adapt, and grow, no matter how many times life knocks you down. Here's her take on it:

1. Can you share an experience where you faced a signifcant challenge or setback in your professional life? How did you handle it, and what strategies did you employ to bounce back from it?

I was employed as a caregiver and I was at work and one of my clients instructed me to give him some of his apple cider so that he could take his medication. And me, following his wishes, I was not informed that he was allergic to apple cider. As the day progressed, my client got so sick we had to call 911 and rush him to the hospital. I was so nervous and upset because I was not aware of his allergies and being a young girl at the time, I was only 15, that scared me so bad because my client had to be rushed to the hospital where he had to be put into the ICU because it was very bad for his abdominal area.

His family was very upset at the service that I was working for, because they had asked for an experienced caregiver. Meanwhile, two weeks later, after he had gotten better and released from the hospital, I was instructed to go back to the client and make sure that I don't give him anything without making sure he was not allergic to it.

After all of that, I made sure that I would not give any of the clients nothing to drink but water, and my theory at the time was, when in doubt, check it out. Meaning, I would have to call the family or the service before I could trust in the client.

2. Resilience often involves maintaining a positive attitude in the face of adversity. Can you discuss a time when you had to deal with a difficult situation at work? How did you maintain and keep a positive outlook during that time?

At the age of 20 years old, I was at work at the time, I was a housekeeper (domestic engineer) and I was proceeding on with my work for the day. I had my headphones on because I love to listen to music and work. About an hour into working, there was a knock on the door. I open the door, and it was my client's mother. My client did not inform her mother that I was an African-American young lady as well as her housekeeper.

She then called the police and I was detained until her daughter came home and let the officers know who I was. I was so embarrassed because I had to sit there, handcuffed and all the neighbors were staring at me, thinking that I was a criminal, and I was only doing my work.

The only thing that helped me through that situation was to think about my son and my daughter that was at home waiting for me. All I could do was to call on the mighty God above and asked Him to take away the evilness and strengthen me to be better than what I was labeled.

3. Adaptability is a key aspect of resilience. Can you provide an example of a situation where you needed to quickly adapt to unexpected changes or obstacles in a project or work environment? How did you approach the situation, and what was the outcome?

About 10 years ago, I arrived at work, and my client was very, very, very sarcastic, crucial and hostile for some unknown reason. I could never get to the bottom of it, but me being me, I had to instantly turn into a mother/social worker/analyzer, and just take on this situation to make some sense of it and also protect myself. Growing up I had a lot of theories that I implanted in my head because I had to figure out things and research a lot of things before I could understand them. So I was really scared because I didn't know how to react to my client but I calmly approached the situation and asked her "are you alright? Is there something that you need to talk about or is there anybody that I can get you to talk to?" She replied in a very hostile way, "No, you don't have to do a damn thing for me."

Now at a very young age, I approached it with one of my theories and as harsh as it may sound, "you have to kill a person with kindness." So as I calmed her down to the best of my ability, I had to really show her that there are better ways to deal with a situation than the way she was trying to deal with it.

She was so upset that she didn't even know what she was upset about!!!! So if I were to respond in a hostile manner to her I would've probably been in jail!!!! So killing it with kindness is the best way to make it easier and better the situation. It's hard but it can be done.

4. Building and maintaining strong relationships can be important in navigating challenging situations. Can you describe a time when you had to collaborate with others to overcome a setback or achieve a common goal? How did you effectively communicate and work with your colleagues to achieve success?

*Maintaining a strong relationship between my coworkers was very hard because there are some of them who like to talk about one another, criticize, and smile in each other's face and act like they really care when they don't. Sometimes when you are put in a situation like that, you really have to be very, very courageous enough to counter react (**give an unexpected or opposite reaction**) with the person or persons, who has the grudge or different opinion on the other (**that they're talking bad about or criticizing**).*

What I had to do was really get to know my coworkers and take them one-on-one and talk to them before I could straighten out the problems that was arising. It wasn't too hard, but it was very very difficult to gather the information to dissect/get into the whole derogatory part of it. So what I had to do is use my strategy that I always use when I'm dealing with my own troubling situations. The majority of the time when I have to conquer a situation or dissect a situation or pry, I would use reverse psychology on them, and it seems to work as long as it's put in the right perspective and that's how I took care of that situation.

5. Resilience often involves learning from failures or mistakes. Can you talk about a specific instance where you encountered failure or made a significant mistake in your work? How did you respond to it, and what did you learn from the experience that helped you grow personally or professionally?

Well I had a really terrible situation at work some years back and sometimes we get to be a little bit of ahead of ourselves and think we know certain things. But every time when you see something, that does not always mean that it is what it seems. I was left a list of instructions to follow at the job which I ignored, thinking it was the same list as normal. I always do things a certain way so I did the same routine that day. As I got ready to leave to go home for the day, something told me I needed to read the list of instructions before I go and low and behold, I had done everything wrong, and I was between a rock and a hard place because I had to be gone by the time the client came home and I had to pick up my children from the daycare. All night all I could do was think of this major catastrophe that I had endured and how I was going to fix it. The next morning, I got a phone call and I was told to report to the dispatch office, and I had to explain what happened and then I had to render the services again and I was not paid for it.

*I took credit for my mistakes, though not proud of it, but the moral of this situation was make sure you follow, the directions clearly before starting a procedure, but **if you mess up, take accountability for your actions. Never assume you know it all, because often times you don't.***

Personal Story #2

This second story of resilience will be from my kid sister, who, like me has had some mental health struggles, but there was also some health issues that she experienced. I will say, when I first was looking for people to write these personal stories, I never thought of interviewing my sister, but I'm glad that I did because I found out a lot of different things about her. My knowledge clearly seemed to rub off on her, LOL!

My sister and I are 2 years apart, she's the younger one (obviously) and we share a lot of the same insight. She was 23 at the time of writing this, so she's definitely wise beyond her years.

1. What coping mechanisms or strategies have you found most helpful in building resilience during difficult times?

*I think just learning yourself first **(specifically your likes, dislikes, triggers, flaws, stressors, etc)** is very important. Only you can know what works for you and not everything works for everyone. Ultimately, you're the only one responsible for your feelings, and for your reactions. For me, some things are writing, taking a breather- that can be staring at the wall for an hour while you try to unscramble your brain. Reading has always helped me, it takes me out of my head and into somewhere else, so does music because you're able to connect with yourself then.*

2. How do you differentiate between healthy coping mechanisms and harmful ones when dealing with mental health struggles?

It's sometimes hard to tell the difference because every situation is not the same. In different situations the roles could be reversed, those previous bad coping mechanisms could be all that could help in the situation. ***A maladaptive coping skill (such as sleeping or overeating) is still a coping skill.***

3. Have you ever experienced a setback in your mental health journey? How did you overcome it, and what lessons did you take away from that experience?

I think everyone experiences at least one major setback in their mental health journey especially when you have a lot on your plate, and you feel like you're in it all alone. I think that's when you must lean on your "support system" the most. When it really comes down to it, you learn who is really there for you annd your wellbeing and which people don't honestly care about your mental. It's also important to make sure you give yourself grace.

4. In your opinion, what role do support networks play in fostering resilience during mental health struggles? How have your relationships with others impacted your ability to bounce back from difficult times?

*Support networks play a huge role in fostering resilience because if you don't have a good one it can set you back and cause more harm than good **(for example, if you have an unsupportive or toxic support network).** I think having someone who knows you better than yourself **(in that moment and can get you out of that black and white thinking)** and having people who are able to listen to you and let you vent is very important. Because in those situations you don't need anyone in your corner who isn't going to validate what you're going through and how you feel.*

5. Have there been moments when you felt like giving up? What motivated you to keep going, and how did you find the strength to persevere?

Thinking about the future, especially if it's something you're passionate about is exciting. It's a huge motivator, and the way I find the strength is just by remembering that the bad doesn't last.

6. How do you maintain a sense of self-compassion and kindness toward yourself when dealing with mental health struggles?

I know I'm a very genuine person and I'm extremely strict and hard on myself so when I'm dealing with those struggles, I try to keep in mind that if I'm not kind to myself how can I expect others to be? Because everything starts with you, if you can't be compassionate to yourself others aren't going to be as willing to extend that same courtesy. Even if it's something as small as giving myself extra time to rest or going on a long drive to clear my head. If I'm taking any small steps to be kind to myself, it still matters.

7. How do you balance the need for self-care with other responsibilities and obligations when you're going through a tough time mentally?

If you don't prioritize yourself, everything else will crumble. I know when things start to get too tough, I make sure I set some time aside to do things I enjoy and take care of myself. For example, if I'm having a tough week at work and school is also kicking my butt, on Saturday I'll sleep in, take myself on a date and just enjoy my company.

8. Looking back on your journey, what advice would you give to someone who is currently struggling with their mental health and seeking to build resilience?

I think my biggest advice is protect your mind **(peace).** *You need to make sure you give yourself grace because you're the only one that must live that life. If anything is weighing too heavy on your mental for too long you need to give it a rest because it's not worth all the damage it can do to you. If you're in a toxic situation and it's constantly getting worse, or you're not feeling valued, DON'T STAY. No one should have to feel unsafe or anxious or just constantly stressing over something they don't have to. If the other party doesn't care enough to notice and change, especially if you make your feelings known and they're not validated, it's not worth it for your sanity.*

Chapter 3: It Starts & Ends with You

"It starts and ends with you" is a profound statement that encapsulates the power of self-awareness, accountability, and personal agency in shaping our lives. It's one of my favorite phrases to tell my clients, especially in coaching. At its core, this phrase speaks to the fundamental truth that our journey of growth, fulfillment, and impact begins within ourselves. It acknowledges that we hold the key to our own happiness, success, and well-being, and emphasizes the importance of taking ownership of our thoughts, actions, and choices. Like my sister said in the previous chapter, you have to really get to know you in order to make sure you're good.

In this chapter, we delve into the significance of this empowering mantra and explore how embracing its wisdom can transform our lives. We will examine the role of self-awareness in understanding our strengths, weaknesses, values, and aspirations, and how this awareness serves as the foundation for personal growth and fulfillment. We will also explore the concept of accountability, acknowledging our responsibility for the outcomes of our lives and the impact of our decisions on ourselves and others.

Furthermore, we will discuss the power of personal agency, recognizing that we have the ability to shape our own destiny and create the life we desire. Through introspection, intentionality, and action, we can align our thoughts, beliefs, and behaviors with our deepest desires and values, ultimately leading to a more authentic and purposeful existence.

Throughout this chapter, we will share insights, reflections, and practical strategies to help you embrace the transformative potential of "it starts and ends with you." By cultivating self-awareness, embracing accountability, and exercising personal agency, you can unleash your full potential, navigate life's challenges with resilience, and create a life of meaning, fulfillment, and impact.

Self-Love is the Key to Life's Greatness

I was listening to Mel Robbins podcast the other day and she was saying that she thinks that confidence is the key to all success. And though I agree with her, but can you be confident without loving yourself? And I'm not talking about the surface level confidence where you are walking into a room full of people, appearing to have it together, while you're dying inside, or maybe I am, and here's why.

I see true confidence as being related to self-love, and my definition of self love is "the belief and respect for oneself to know that anything you want is possible, but also to be able to walk away from situations that don't serve you." So if I'm about to do a public speaking gig in front of a room full of people, I might still get anxiety, but I also don't have to fake it till I make it, because I actually believe I can do it.

I'm not faking confidence, there's no self doubt, but that doesn't mean that I'm not gonna be a little scared. Especially if it's something that I've never done before or a topic I've never spoken about before. In fact, sometimes I get the most anxious about things I'm truly passionate about because I want to get my point across effectively. And you know sometimes when you're too excited about something, and you nerd out and start rambling off on a tangent. Yeah, that's me, when it comes to anything mental health, self love, or wellbeing related. So again, lack of confidence isn't the problem. The anxiety I feel is actually excitement about the fact I get to talk about my passion for x amount of minutes.

Can confidence even be enough to get you through in the first place?

I truly don't think so.

Not to say that Mel Robbins or any other confidence coach or social media guru got it wrong, I just feel like they missed a step. True confidence starts with self love.

If you're able to have enough self-love, you automatically are more confident, you have more self-respect, you practice good boundaries, you're in healthy relationships because you know when to walk away, you most likely don't stay in one sided relationships for very long. But even if you're not completely confident in your abilities because you're trying something new, you still love yourself enough to try it anyways.

Self-love is the foundation of a fulfilling and authentic life, rooted in the acceptance and appreciation of your true self. It means recognizing your inherent worth, valuing your strengths, and embracing your imperfections without judgment. Self-love involves prioritizing your well-being, setting healthy boundaries, and making choices that align with your values and goals. It is the act of showing yourself the kindness, compassion, and forgiveness you so readily offer others. Ultimately, self-love empowers you to navigate life with confidence, resilience, and a deep sense of inner peace, knowing you are deserving of love and respect just as as you are.

Confidence is often situational—it comes from external achievements, skills, or validation, and can fluctuate based on circumstances. However, self-love is deeply rooted and unconditional. It provides a stable foundation for success because it fuels resilience, self-worth, and intrinsic motivation.

When you love yourself, you're more likely to take risks, pursue your dreams, and recover from setbacks because your sense of value doesn't depend on external factors. Self-love encourages self-awareness, which helps you align your goals with your true desires rather than societal expectations. Confidence may help you perform well in the moment, but self-love ensures that you continue to grow and thrive over the long term, even in the face of challenges. Self-love is the internal engine that drives authentic and sustainable success. In fact, any time that people have argued and claimed to have self-love, especially in therapy and coaching sessions, we would dig a little deeper and realize that at some point, they had lessened their level of self-love/self-respect and allowed themselves to put someone else first which can lead to people pleasing; which we will save for another chapter.

This chapter simply builds off the previous chapters about resilience, but it also focuses more on the journey instead of simply the destination. The biggest lesson 2024 taught me was that self-development is a journey, you never stop learning about yourself and trying to love yourself and improve.

I was someone who struggled and suffered in silence with mental health for my entire teenage years into young adulthood until last year (2023). During my journey, there were points I was suicidal and wanted to end it all, yet would still smile behind all the pain. I had gone through toxic relationships and countless other things (within relationships which is a completely other book someday) that caused me to be so broken. But now I am a woman of God who has come out on the other end of all that, still believing there is good, still believing in God, still wanting to help people because no one was there to help me through my struggle. Who knows though, confidence might be the key to success for you and that's great. No one's wrong for it, we all want the same thing and are getting to the same place, the point here is that it all starts and ends with you.

My reality is that no one could save me because I had to be willing to save myself first. I had to look deep within and realize that I was worthy just as I am, and I deserved more than what I was allowing from the men I associated with. I allowed them to treat me as if I worth less than I was, because I felt worthless. I felt like I had no value, and that I needed a man for validation. It took me accepting myself and truly embodying and loving the skin that I'm in, even if I never become thinner or get the clear skin or xyz, because that would mean my confidence was conditional. And that's not what I wanted. I needed to be loved unconditionally, and the only person that could truly offer that to me other than

God, was my self.

So the following chapter is a tribute to you and your journey thus far. I hope that it encourages you and helps you to realize that you are worthy just as you are. You're not broken, you're not damaged goods, you're not some self-improvement project that has to become your highest self before you're worthy, you are worthy NOW. You deserve a place on this earth, and just because something bad happened to you that doesn't mean it has to be the end of your story.

You are a woman (black, white, Asian, or Middle Eastern), and you are resilient and will get through this. You are powerful, you go through a literal period of bleeding for 3-7 days every month and you are survive it (prayerfully). Some of us have even given birth or had the luxury to conceive, and whether the baby made it full term or not, there was only a 20% chance that you would even conceive.

You are a miracle, you're God's masterpiece, your life is worth it, you are loved, you are amazing, you are valued. I love you, I don't even have to know you to love you. I love you simply because I see the potential in you. I see your greatness. You wouldn't have picked up a book called "Radiate: Unleash Your Inner Light" and came this far to not be a greatness. And you're not a masterpiece in the making or a millionaire in the making or anything "in the making", you are everything that you will ever need to be right now. Once you learn to accept yourself just as you are, in the present moment, that's when life begins to take a whole new turn.

Remember, self-love is a foundational pillar of wellbeing and personal growth, encompassing acceptance, compassion, and nurturing towards oneself. Its importance cannot be overstated, as it forms the basis for healthy relationships, resilience in the face of adversity, and fulfillment in life. Here's the role self-love can actually play in your life:

1. Enhanced Mental Health: Self-love promotes positive mental health by fostering a sense of self-worth and acceptance. When you love yourself, you are more likely to practice self-care, set healthy boundaries, and prioritize your well-being. This can lead to reduced stress, anxiety, and depression, as well as greater overall psychological resilience.

2. Healthy Relationships: Loving yourself sets the standard for how you allow others to treat you. When you have a strong sense of self-love, you are less likely to tolerate mistreatment or settle for less than you deserve in relationships. Moreover, self-love allows you to give and receive love authentically, fostering deeper connections with others based on mutual respect and appreciation. When you love yourself first, you set a standard for how you want to be treated and nothing less.

3. Resilience and Self-Compassion: Self-love provides a buffer against life's challenges by fostering resilience and self-compassion. When you love yourself, you are better equipped to navigate setbacks, failures, and disappointments with kindness and understanding. Rather than berating yourself for mistakes, self-love allows you to acknowledge your humanity and learn from experiences without judgment.

4. Personal Growth and Fulfillment: Embracing self-love is essential for personal growth and fulfillment. It empowers you to pursue your passions, goals, and aspirations with confidence and conviction. When you love yourself, you believe in your inherent worth and potential, fueling a sense of purpose and motivation to live authentically and pursue your dreams.

5. Authenticity and Empowerment: Self-love encourages authenticity and empowers you to live according to your values and beliefs. It allows you to embrace your unique qualities, quirks, and imperfections without seeking validation or approval from others. By honoring your true self, you cultivate a sense of empowerment and autonomy in navigating life's choices and challenges.

In essence, self-love is the cornerstone of a fulfilling and meaningful life. It is a journey of self-discovery and self-acceptance that yields profound rewards, enabling you to live life with greater joy, purpose, and fulfillment.

Any coaching or therapy, or additional services that you receive are simply resources. No one can make you change or change for you, you have to be willing to do the work. I've had so many clients that come to therapy wanting a different life and expecting me to fix them, but if they don't want to actually take things seriously and actually do the work, they won't get anywhere. We'll just end up in a hamster wheel, having the same meaningless conversations over and over again. At some point, you have to want more for yourself.

Controlling your own reality is about recognizing the power you have to shape your experiences, perceptions, and outcomes in life. While you may not have control over external events or circumstances, you do have control over how you respond to them and the meaning you assign to them. Here's how you can take control of your own reality, if you haven't already:

1. Mindset: Your mindset plays a crucial role in shaping your reality. By adopting a positive and growth-oriented mindset, you can reframe challenges as opportunities for learning and growth. Instead of dwelling on setbacks or limitations, focus on what you can control and how you can overcome obstacles with resilience and determination.

2. Perception: Your perception of reality is influenced by your beliefs, attitudes, and interpretations of events. By cultivating awareness of your thoughts and biases, you can choose to view situations from a more empowering perspective. Shift your focus from what you lack to what you have, from problems to solutions, and from fear to possibility.

3. Intention: Setting clear intentions allows you to align your thoughts, actions, and energy with your desired outcomes. By defining what you want to create or achieve, you can direct your attention and efforts towards manifesting your goals. Visualize success, affirm your intentions, and take inspired action to bring your vision into reality.

4. Choice: You always have the power to choose how you respond to any given situation. Instead of reacting impulsively or passively accepting circumstances, consciously choose your thoughts, words, and actions. Take ownership of your decisions and their consequences, recognizing that each choice you make shapes your reality.

5. Focus: Where you direct your attention determines your reality. By focusing on what you want to manifest rather than what you want to avoid, you can attract positive outcomes and opportunities into your life. Cultivate gratitude, appreciation, and mindfulness to amplify the positive aspects of your reality and minimize negativity.

6. Action: Your actions are the building blocks of your reality. By taking intentional and consistent action towards your goals, you can create the life you desire. Break down your goals into manageable steps, prioritize tasks based on their importance and urgency, and persist in the face of challenges or setbacks.

7. Adaptability: Flexibility and adaptability are essential for navigating the ever-changing landscape of reality. Embrace uncertainty as a natural part of life and remain open to new possibilities and opportunities. Adjust your plans and strategies as needed, staying resilient and resourceful in the face of unexpected events.

Ultimately, controlling your own reality is about recognizing the power you have to influence your experiences and shape the course of your life. By cultivating a positive mindset, intentional focus, and empowered action, you can create a reality that aligns with your values, aspirations, and dreams.

Chapter 4: Discovering YourTrue Self

In the journey of life, amidst the chaos of daily routines and societal expectations, there exists a profound quest that resonates within each of us – the quest to discover our true selves. This pursuit is not merely a fleeting desire for self-improvement but a fundamental need to uncover the essence of who we are, beneath the layers of conditioning, expectations, and external influences. In this chapter, we delve into the significance of discovering our true selves and the transformative power it holds in shaping our lives.

At its core, discovering our true self involves peeling back the layers of societal norms, cultural conditioning, and past experiences to reveal the authentic essence of our being. It is about reconnecting with our deepest desires, passions, values, and strengths that define us at our core. While this journey may seem daunting or uncertain, it is an essential step towards living a life of authenticity, fulfillment, and purpose. I have a whole 8-week program just on self-discovery within my coaching brand.

In a world that often encourages conformity and uniformity, embracing our true selves is an act of rebellion – a declaration of our inherent worth and uniqueness. It is a reclaiming of our individuality, free from the constraints of external expectations or judgments. By embarking on this journey of self-discovery, we reclaim the power to shape our own narrative, forge our own path, and live life on our own terms.

Moreover, discovering our true selves is not just an individual pursuit but a collective endeavor with far-reaching implications. As we uncover our authentic selves, we become catalysts for positive change in the world around us. Our actions, fueled by clarity of purpose and alignment with our values, have the potential to inspire others, cultivate meaningful connections, and contribute to a more authentic and compassionate society.

Throughout this chapter, we will explore various aspects of self-discovery, from the importance of introspection and self-awareness to practical strategies for uncovering our true selves. We will delve into the challenges and rewards of this journey, offering insights, reflections, and exercises to guide you along the path towards greater authenticity and self-fulfillment.

Ultimately, the journey of discovering our true selves is a deeply personal and transformative odyssey – a journey of self-discovery that leads us home to ourselves. It is a journey worth embarking on, for in the depths of our true selves lies the key to unlocking our fullest potential and living a life of purpose, passion, and authenticity.

How is this chapter different from the previous chapter?

Last chapter was about how it starts and ends with you. It was meant to inspire and to motivate you, think of it as the pre-workout. The stretch before you hop on the treadmill, but now it's go-time babe. This next chapter is about you actually going full-speed towards the target. But what is the target? Why are you reading this book? What inner light are you trying to unleash? How do you do that? So many questions, but don't worry, they'll be answered, at least partially.

The biggest thing to remember though is that self-development is a lifelong journey, it's not like you just read one self-help book and boom you're healed now. Or maybe it is if you actually do the work in this book, and move forward everyday with self-love, self-respect, and self-assurance. That's all you really need.

The Journey of Self-Discovery

We all know that the hardest part of any journey is the beginning. You have to be willing to trust the process, stay consistent, and continue to work hard until the process becomes easier. No, not easier, but more of a routine, because growth is never easy or necessarily pleasant. I just recently finished writing my chapter for the Becoming an Unstoppable Woman: Mompreneur edition book which will be out before this one (so go pick that up as well) and I realized that it's not supposed to be easy.

I went from feeling a lack of confidence about writing and finishing this book, to signing up to co-author a second book, and planning to write several other books. Thinking generally of the book "The Mountain is You", it is helpful to note that once you get past the initial hesitation, you realize that the horizon is actually more beautiful from the top. But you would've never known if you didn't take that first step, and keep climbing Mt. You.

We are capable of so much and meant to do so much in this life, but if we never get the confidence to take the journey, we'll miss out on all of life's offerings.

The purpose that you were given, your reason for being on this earth and for continuing to live each day is never supposed to be easy, because it's personalized to you. There's no manual, ebook, or course that can tell you "how to life" (and if there is they're lying) because everyone was meant to go on different journeys for a reason. The hard work, the pain, the hurt, all of the bad that we encounter, is a necessary evil on this journey. Your story is so much better with the scars and bruises that were healed. It makes us more grateful and motivated to continue because we remember where we came from and how far we have come.

And if you do get stuck and need help along the way, don't be afraid to reach out to your support systems for help. You can also always reach out to me at @uniquetransfhermations on Instagram and schedule a free discovery call so that we can work on creating your life's manual together. A program or course that best fits you and your journey. I'll be your partner and you'll be the tour guide, as we embark into open waters.

Don't get discouraged, keep going.

Journal Prompt

These questions can be answered in any order and will help you start your journey towards self-discovery. Choose one question to start off with and take about 10 minutes to get clear and concise about your answers.

Getting to Know Myself

1. *"My definition of success is _ _ _ _ _ _ _ _ _ _"*
2. *A day in my dream lifestyle would include*
3. *What are my core values and beliefs, and how do they guide my decisions and actions?*
4. *Do my core values and beliefs align with what I am currently doing with my life? Why or why not?*
5. *What are my top 3 long-term goals? (Next 5 to 10 years, lifetime achievement goals)*
6. *What are my top 5 short-term goals? (Think 3 to 6 months, a year max)*
7. *Is my current lifestyle getting me closer or farther away from the woman I want to become?*
8. *What hobbies or activities make me lose track of time and bring me pure joy?*
9. *How do I handle or cope with stress and difficult situations, and what can I learn from it?*
10. *What patterns or habits have helped me in the past, but are no longer serving me?*

Passion vs Purpose Explained

Passion and purpose are closely related but distinct concepts, so let's go into it:

Passion refers to intense enthusiasm or strong emotions toward something. It's the driving force that fuels your interests, motivates you to pursue certain activities, and brings you joy and fulfillment. Passion often involves activities or pursuits that you deeply enjoy and find meaningful.

Purpose, on the other hand, relates to the reason why you exist or the contribution you want to make to the world. It's the overarching goal or direction that guides your actions and decisions. Purpose gives your life meaning and helps you understand the significance of your actions in the grand scheme of things.

In essence, passion is more about what excites you and brings you joy in the present moment, while purpose is about the broader impact you want to have on the world and the legacy you want to leave behind. Passion can contribute to fulfilling your purpose, as it often drives you to engage in activities that align with your larger goals and values. However, purpose provides a deeper sense of meaning and direction that goes beyond personal interests and desires. This is why you can have multiple passions, but typically only have one purpose in life.

What is your why?

We all have a reason that we get up every morning and go to our jobs, and even leave the house every day. I believe the world can be split into three types of people. For some of us, we enjoy life and are excited to go through life everyday (we're like the Spongebobs of the world). Then there's others who get up everyday out of necessity, whether it's because we have kids or maybe we're the one that pay bills or we're made to feel as though we have no other choice (by society or sometimes our own parents/family members). But for others, they might not have a reason for getting up every morning, or might not know why they were sent to earth.

There is a percentage of people that are getting up every reason and going about their life, monotonously, dreading life, living every day with no purpose. It's heartbreaking, but I know this because I was one of these people. But now I'm more of a mixture of category 1 and 2. I get up everyday because I have to as a mother, and head of household, but I also enjoy getting up. Now don't get me wrong, I still have my days where I wake up and I don't feel like doing anything and I get discouraged, but that's now only 1 to 2 days out of the week max, as compared to every single day. I've come to learn that my purpose is to help others become healed enough and empowered enough to fulfill their own purposes. It is to help people achieve "self-transcendence".

There was an updated version of Maslow's hierarchy of needs that I came across or was introduced to back in college, that included self-transcendence. According to Britannica, "self-actualization, in psychology, a concept regarding the process by which an individual reaches his or her full potential." Maslow's updated hierarchy includes self-transcendence which comes after self-actualization, and is basically having a "sense of meaning and purpose" in ones life.

So anyone that I coach, see for therapy, or come across in daily life, I am always working with them to not only see their full potential, but to live a more purposeful, rich and meaningful life. And I understand that I cannot force people to do things that they aren't ready for, but I also believe that everyone is meant for greater. Sometimes having that belief is enough, at least for the moment, because it keeps you going when you know that there's something bigger to look forward to. I get all doom and gloom when I think about the fact that some people won't change and that the world is a terrible place, so I choose not to think like that. I'm not able to work at my full capacity as a Negative Nancy, so I choose to be Radiant Rae, the positive one who sees life as being full of lessons and experiences and looks forward to new days.

So really quickly, I'm going to give you all a brief journal prompt that is going to help you figure out how to find your passion.

Journal Prompt

Answering these 10 questions will help you start thinking about the possibilities for the things that you are passionate about, and help you develop a purpose.

1. *What was your favorite thing to do growing up?*
2. *If money were no object, how would you choose to spend your time?*
3. *When you were a child, what did you dream of doing when you grew up? Why did you let go of that dream? Is it still possible?*
4. *What topics are most eager to talk about/learn more about?*
5. *What would you do with your life if you had a guarantee of success?*
6. *What are you good at? What do others often compliment you on?*
7. *If you could solve one problem in the world, what would it be?*
8. *What would you do with your life if you had no fear?*
9. *When do you feel the most energized and alive?*
10. *What do you value most in life? How can you align your passion with your values?*

How do we get there?

Developing your purpose in life is a deeply personal journey that often begins with self-reflection. It involves taking the time to explore your interests, values, strengths, and dreams. By asking yourself probing questions such as "What activities bring me joy and fulfillment?" or "What do I truly value in life?", you can start to gain clarity on what matters most to you. This introspection lays the foundation for understanding your unique path forward.

Identifying your talents and strengths is another essential step in developing your purpose. Take stock of your natural abilities and the things you excel at. Whether it's problem-solving, creativity, leadership, or empathy, recognizing your strengths can provide valuable insights into potential avenues for pursuing your purpose.

Setting meaningful goals aligned with your values and passions can give your life direction and purpose. Think about what you want to achieve in various aspects of your life, such as your career, relationships, personal growth, and community involvement. These goals serve as guiding beacons, helping you stay focused and motivated as you navigate your journey.

Exploring your interests and being open to new experiences is key to uncovering your purpose. Cultivate curiosity and embrace opportunities that spark your enthusiasm. Whether it's trying out new hobbies, embarking on adventures, or delving into topics that intrigue you, each experience can offer valuable insights into what resonates most deeply with you.

Finding ways to contribute to the world around you can also play a significant role in shaping your sense of purpose. Whether through volunteering, activism, mentorship, or creative expression, making a positive impact can provide a profound sense of fulfillment and meaning. Consider how you can leverage your skills and passions to contribute to causes that align with your values.

Embracing growth and adaptability is essential as you navigate your journey toward discovering your purpose. Understand that your sense of purpose may evolve over time as you learn and grow. Stay open to new possibilities and opportunities for personal and professional development that resonate with your values and aspirations.

Listening to your intuition and trusting your inner wisdom can guide you along your path to purpose. Pay attention to the moments when you feel most alive and aligned with your true self. These moments of clarity can offer valuable insights into your purpose and direction in life.

By engaging in self-reflection, identifying your strengths, setting meaningful goals, exploring your interests, contributing to the world, embracing growth, and trusting your intuition, you can develop a deeper sense of purpose and fulfillment in your life. Remember that your purpose is unique to you and may unfold gradually over time, so embrace the journey with patience and openness.

Addressing limiting beliefs

Addressing limiting beliefs involves a multi-step process aimed at fostering self-awareness and promoting personal growth. Initially, it's crucial to pinpoint the specific thoughts or beliefs that are holding you back. These beliefs often manifest as self-critical or negative thoughts about yourself, your abilities, or your potential. By recognizing these patterns, you can begin to understand the areas where you might be limiting yourself.

Limiting beliefs often find their roots in the external environment, influenced by societal norms, cultural expectations, upbringing, and past experiences. Society sets standards dictating how we should look, behave, and succeed, creating pressure to conform and fostering beliefs that constrain our individuality and potential. Family dynamics, including parental expectations and modeling behavior, significantly shape our perceptions of ourselves and our abilities. For example, an upbringing where failure is stigmatized or success is narrowly defined can lead to beliefs that limit our confidence and aspirations.

Educational environments also play a pivotal role in shaping beliefs about intelligence, academic abilities, and potential for success. Standardized testing, grading systems, and comparisons with peers can reinforce beliefs about our capabilities and limit our academic or career aspirations. Media, including advertising and social media, perpetuates unrealistic standards of beauty, success, and happiness, fostering feelings of inadequacy or unworthiness through constant exposure to idealized images and lifestyles.

Peer influences and social dynamics further contribute to the formation of limiting beliefs. The desire for acceptance and fear of rejection often lead to conforming to perceived norms and beliefs about what is achievable or acceptable. Negative experiences of criticism or rejection from peers can reinforce feelings of insecurity and limit our sense of self-worth. Overall, external influences play a significant role in shaping our beliefs about ourselves and our potential. Recognizing these influences is the first step towards challenging and overcoming limiting beliefs, empowering us to embrace our full potential and pursue our aspirations with confidence and resilience.

One example of a limiting belief developed from society is the notion that success is solely determined by external factors such as wealth, status, or recognition. In many cultures, there's a prevailing belief that one must achieve certain milestones or meet specific societal standards to be considered successful. This can lead individuals to internalize the idea that their worth and value are tied solely to external achievements, such as their job title, salary, or material possessions.

Once identified, it's important to question the validity of these limiting beliefs. Challenge yourself to consider whether there is concrete evidence supporting these beliefs or if they are based on outdated assumptions or past experiences. This step involves exploring alternative perspectives and possibilities, allowing you to broaden your mindset and challenge entrenched negative thinking patterns.

Understanding the origins of your limiting beliefs is another essential aspect of the process. Reflect on the experiences, societal influences, or comparisons to others that may have contributed to the formation of these beliefs. By gaining insight into their roots, you can develop greater empathy and understanding for yourself, paving the way for constructive self-reflection and growth.

Reframing the narrative is a powerful technique for overcoming limiting beliefs. Replace negative thoughts with empowering and realistic alternatives that affirm your strengths, capabilities, and potential. By consciously choosing to focus on positive affirmations, you can gradually shift your mindset and cultivate a more optimistic outlook on yourself and your abilities.

Stepping outside your comfort zone is an effective way to challenge limiting beliefs and build self-confidence. Engage in activities or tasks that contradict your negative beliefs, providing tangible evidence of your capabilities and potential for growth. Embrace these opportunities to celebrate your successes and reinforce positive self-beliefs through firsthand experiences.

Throughout this process, practicing self-compassion is essential. Be kind and patient with yourself as you work to overcome limiting beliefs. Recognize that change takes time and effort, and allow yourself to make mistakes along the way. Cultivating a sense of self-compassion can help you navigate challenges with greater resilience and perseverance.

Seeking support from trusted friends, family members, mentors, or professionals can provide invaluable encouragement and guidance. Sharing your struggles with others can offer fresh perspectives and reinforce your efforts to overcome limiting beliefs. Surround yourself with a supportive network that believes in your potential and encourages your personal growth journey.

Addressing limiting beliefs is an ongoing endeavor that requires consistency and perseverance. Stay committed to challenging negative thoughts and replacing them with positive affirmations. Celebrate your progress, no matter how small, and remain focused on your journey toward self-growth and empowerment. With dedication and determination, you can break free from self-imposed barriers and cultivate a mindset that supports your overall well-being and fulfillment.

When we work through our limiting beliefs, we allow ourselves to dream a little bigger, and make room for things that we initially didn't think were possible. It allows us to become the women we are meant to be.

Self-Love & Spirituality

Starting in 2023, I started to take my relationship with God more seriously. Even though I was raised Christian and went to church because of my grandparents, I never really had my own relationship with God. And now, to be transparent, I still don't fully know what that looks like, but I have come a lot closer than I was years before. I'm at least making an attempt to become more disciplined and less worldly, even though I'm not perfect. I never really was one that would cuss or twerk, or smoke or drink too heavily. So when starting my spiritual journey, those things were easy to quit.

My biggest sin was always fornication. It was something I always knew I should save for marriage, but never did. I ended up having a baby out of wedlock at 25 and that was when I realized that things really needed to change. Having my son made me realize that I wanted to be even more intentional about myself as well as my spiritual journey and becoming more disciplined. I realized that I had been giving my body, my heart, my mind to people that didn't deserve me. The worst part was that I knew they didn't while I was dealing with them, but I was still allowing it.

And then one day, I realized that the reason that I was allowing it was because I felt like I deserved it. I was so desperate to wanted by someone, even superficially and then I didn't truly desire them. The realization came one night when I called a friend while contemplating a link up with an on-again, off-again "ex", if we can even call him that. "Why are you on the fence about it?" My friend asked.

"I'm not on the fence about it, it's really an easy decision, I'm just making it hard."

"Well stop making it hard then."

UH DUH! PSYCHOLOGY 101! Why was I making a big deal out of a no-brainer?! The answer was simple, don't let him come over then. Case closed.

So I didn't. But then I was going to let someone else come over and chill, with the intention just to talk and hang out, but I ended up deading that too. I also quit talking on the phone with the other people I was having a conversation with and turned both phones on DND and told everybody I was going to sleep. I'm telling y'all, I was so desperate to just be in somebody's company, but it's like why? They don't deserve to be around me, and half of the time, they're a lame anyways. Why am I wasting my time?

As I proceeded to get in the shower and do my nightly routine, I had on some gospel music. I don't know about y'all, but whenever I listen to gospel music, that's the time that I heard God speaking to me the

the most, or at least it seems like it. During my shower, I thought about the events of that night. After deciding not to have the "ex" come over and turning the phone on DND, he had FaceTimed me twice, so I called him back. I hesitated explaining the truth to him, but since I had been trying to get better at communication, I just went ahead. I told him that I couldn't allow myself to keep going down this road with him, and that if he couldn't take me seriously in the way that I wanted, then I needed him to just leave me alone.

At first he protested, claiming he did take me serious and just needed time before we would be in a relationship again, but after continuing to plead my case, and not letting up, he finally relented, "Alright, well just text me," he stated before we got off the phone. 'Just text me' was something he'd always say before we'd stop talking to each other because he knows that I don't like texting.

"Okay," I said, before hanging up, again knowing full well I wouldn't text him. I knew that this meant the end of us, for good this time. But for some reason, replaying this conversation in the shower, I wasn't as sad as I normally was. I mean yeah I was sad because I was letting my favorite "good time" go, but I wasn't in tears sad or even depressed like usual.

I thought to myself and this is where I think God was talking to me, so let's just go with it, *no one ever said being disciplined is easy. No one ever said self-love was easy. Sometimes choosing ourselves is the hardest decision that we have to make. No one ever said doing the right thing was easy, but it's still the right thing.*

I know it was God because I have never said something like that to myself before. I don't even talk to myself that way. But it was just what I needed to hear. God knew I needed to hear that, because you know what, after my shower, I was okay.

I didn't fall into a depressive state like I normally would've, I got out, made my son his bottle, turned on the TV, and ate some snacks. Kept both phones on DND and stayed strong.

This story is so huge for me because it's something I never would've been able to do before taking my self love journey seriously. The "ex" in question was my fave "spin-the-blocker" as I called him, we always had a good time whenever we linked, but it was purely physical, and as much as we tried to deny it, we both knew that.

Ironically enough, I had listened to a podcast episode before the shower by The Self Love Fix called "Expectations vs Standards and the impact of BOTH on your love life". And she was talking about how standards should be unwavering, and if they waver, they're not standards. And this is so true because I expect to be treated better and respected, but when it actually comes down to it, I always fold, and lead with my body, rather than with my mind. I was definitely always ego-led like she had said, because I could easily make someone do what I wanted by manipulating them into a relationship so that I wouldn't feel bad about fornication because "at least they're my boyfriend." The anxious state she was talking about definitely hit different for me.

And I wanted to stop being manipulative. Not only that, but my best friend had told me earlier that week that I was toxic in a relationship. And though offended, I admitted that I had been playing a game with men, and that it was very toxic, and I wanted to stop that.

I know that God was changing me, working on me ever so slowly, because before, I wouldn't have cared about my intentions towards people, I would have been very self-serving in any way I needed to be and never apologized for it, but that's not the way that God designed us.

I've always been a reckless girl, not in a dangerous way, but just in a "do what makes you happy" sort of way, which only was reckless sexually. So part of learning to love myself was realizing that if I wanted men to take me serious, I had to take myself serious and get clear about my standards. I needed to stand on business, like I was always telling my clients to do. If I wanted a God-fearing man who actually wanted marriage and was going to respect me and if I wanted to make the relationship last more than just a few months, I needed to stop settling for less.

I tell my clients all the time that they need to "stand on business" and be true to who they are, but I wasn't even doing it. Listen, a part of me wanted to leave this chapter out, but then it wouldn't be telling my true story, and I'm all about authenticity.

Tools for Self-Reflection

A really great tool that I learned that night by listening to the Therapy for Black Girls podcast is "to analyze your needs and wants from a relationship". This is something that I had to do in my head, when I was telling my fave spend-the-blocker that I couldn't continue to pursue things with him anymore. "We're not compatible," I'd said.

"But we are compatible, that's why we were in a relationship before," he stated.

Which was true, but cheating was always an issue for him. I brought up to him that getting cheated on and being played with was something that I couldn't go through with him again and that's when he said to just text him.

This was me standing up for myself, about how I needed more than what he was offering me, and that despite him thinking that he was taking me seriously, he actually wasn't, because there would always be someone else. So take a minute, and think about your current relationship, situationship, or your previous relationship, if you're single.

Is this something that you want? Some of us want to be in a situationship because it's all we have time for. But even then, is that really what we want long-term? Even if we say it is, because I was that girl too, it's a protective mechanism, and often times we want to be someone's girl, we just don't want to get played with. And that's okay, but be honest about what you really want from a man and why?

Go a step further and even figure out what you need. Consider your needs being your non-negotiables. Things that your ideal man will do without question. These needs don't have to be in any particular order right now, but eventually, they'll become your standards. And the wants are your expectations.

My Wants and Needs List

Wants

–I want flowers. It doesn't have to be everyday, but at least once or twice a month, just because.

–I want him to be spontaneous. This is almost a need because in my opinion spontaneity makes the relationship more fun, but it's also not important enough to be a standard.

–I want him to enjoy reading. It's nice to have a man that's smart, but there's also other ways to gain knowledge. I'd just like him to enjoy learning.

–He only smokes or drinks occasionally. I don't want an alcoholic or a pothead.

–I want him to rub my feet.

–I want him to be business minded. He doesn't have to be, at least at first because I feel like it's something that I'll naturally bring out of him, but he can't want to work for someone else forever, unless he has an amazingly paid job.

–He can't want to be stuck where he's at. He has to be open to moving somewhere else. It's not really a standard though because it'll eventually change.

–Likes seafood.

–Likes watching movies.

Needs

-He has to be God fearing and truly in his Bible. Prayer needs to be a regular practice.

-He has to value me, my feelings, and my opinion.

-He has to want growth and be driven.

-He has to dress nice.

-He has to be nice to me.

-He has to listen to me. I love having me a man that is also my Bestfriend.

-He has to have his own money and be willing to spend it. I don't like when men ask me to pay for stuff, it's just not attractive.

-He has to have some level of intelligence, even if he's not a college graduate.

-He has to be funny. He has to make me laugh.

-We have to be compatible, which means that we have to have the roughly same goals in life.

-I need a man that knows how to communicate. Someone who knows the importance of telling me his problems instead of shutting me out or going ghost on me, and is also willing to hear my problems and isn't going to just brush me off.

-He has to want marriage, he has to want to have at least one other kid, and he has to be willing to accept my son.

 -He has to have a good paying job. He needs to make $20 an hour minimum.

-He has to have a car and.a license. The two don't always coexist.

-He can't live with his mom. (I like older men and there's no reason 30 year olds should still be living with their momma).

-He can't have more than 1 other kid. I only have 1 so it only makes sense.

-We have to go on a date, at least once or twice a week.

-Communication is key. I want to get a phone call at least once a day, even if it's only for 15 minutes and texts throughout the day.

-He has to be affectionate.

-He has to be attentive to me and considerate. I don't want an aggressive or nonchalant man.

-He has to take initiative. I love a man who leads and who's direct. I don't like when men beat around the bush.

-He has to make me want to be better. I want to be able to learn from him, that's what partnership is all about.

-I have to respect him.

-I have to find him attractive. I don't care if it's shallow, I want cute kids and I want to be happily married, attraction matters.

-He doesn't smoke cigarettes.

-He likes to show me off.

-He has to be understanding.

-He has to contribute to my life and add value, other than just financially or sexually.

-He has to be open-minded and willing to try new things.

Doing that for the first time, I realized that I had way more needs (standards) than I did wants (expectations) which makes sense. There should be more standards than expectations, simply because even if someone doesn't meet our expectations, we want them to be able to still make us happy by meeting our standards. I actually encourage you to take a moment and do this wants and needs list for what you expect out of life as well. I find that it'll be really helpful to get clear about that because then you will be have more clarity on a direction.

Reframing the Loneliness

Once I took inventory of my wants and needs, I took a good look at my "roster" which wasn't very much of a roster at all, only included a few exes. I realized that none of them fit the requirements for what I was looking for. Truth be told, it was my fault because I didn't value myself, let alone have a clue what I wanted. I was just dating aimlessly, hoping to figure it out as I went along. But I couldn't do that once I developed standards. *Where do I go from here?* I asked myself, fully knowing good and well the answer.

It meant being single. Single, but never lonely, because I'd be working on myself until the right man came around. Taking myself on dates and getting to know myself, and developing self love so that when the right one came along, I was actually ready for him. I wanted to healed and healthy in a relationship versus my old ways as broken and toxic. A lot of us as women don't want to admit it, but we are the problem and sometimes cause the relationship to go left. There was a few times I let my entitlement as a woman get the best of me, and it was a reason that I let a good man go.

Hindsight is always 20/20 and I was definitely a problem, 99% of the time. I had a disgustingly ugly attitude and an extreme distrust for men which had started in childhood and I should've never even been in relationships in the first place. I was the epitome of an angry black woman as a teenager, and I didn't care. My favorite lines were "oh well" or "I don't care" when someone would call me mean or rude. There was a lot of hurt and damage that I went through in my childhood, and being angry just seemed easier than talking about it. I also can admit that my mother was not the most healed human being (no offense mom), but I just felt like I could do whatever I wanted.

Let me clear the air though, my mother and grandmother are both great women and they did the best that they could, but the reality is that hurt people, hurt people. My grandma did the best to pour into us and make us feel loved while my mom was busy working all the time as a single mother. But they both had traumatic childhoods and lives which you read about in the first few chapters. So I had to heal myself if I ever wanted to be in a healthy relationship, and get married. Plus, I was a mom and I wanted to be healed for my son.

Embracing Your Uniqueness

Embracing your uniqueness involves a journey of self-discovery and acceptance, rooted in deep self-awareness. Take the time to understand yourself, reflecting on your strengths, weaknesses, values, and passions. Through this introspection, you can recognize the distinct qualities and experiences that shape your identity and set you apart from others.

Acceptance is a fundamental aspect of embracing your uniqueness. Embrace both the positive and negative aspects of yourself, understanding that nobody is perfect. By accepting your imperfections and quirks, you pave the way for self-love and personal growth.

Rather than comparing yourself to others, celebrate what makes you unique. Focus on your individuality and the characteristics that make you stand out. Reject the pressure to conform to societal norms or expectations, and instead, embrace your authenticity.

Your life story is a tapestry of experiences that have shaped who you are today. Own your journey, including both the triumphs and challenges. Embrace your past and the lessons it has taught you, sharing your story authentically with others.

Find ways to express yourself authentically, whether through art, writing, music, fashion, or any other form of creativity. Allow your personality to shine through, unapologetically showcasing what makes you unique.

Surround yourself with positivity by seeking out supportive individuals who appreciate and celebrate your uniqueness. Distance yourself from those who try to change you or make you feel inadequate, prioritizing relationships that uplift and inspire you.

Challenge yourself to step out of your comfort zone and pursue your interests and passions, even if they may seem unconventional. Embracing new opportunities and taking risks can lead to further self-discovery and growth.

Above all, practice self-love and compassion. Treat yourself with kindness and respect, prioritizing your physical, mental, and emotional well-being. Remember that you are worthy of love and acceptance just as you are, and embrace your uniqueness with pride.

I've developed a life-story coaching program titled "The Birth of a Woman" which is a 9-week coaching program to help you reframe different stages of your life. As we are in utero for 9 months (although it is 40 weeks), the course is meant to take you through a sort of rebirthing process, allowing you to accept the things you can't change, and change the things you can. At the end of the program, you will write a sort of manifesto, to help you gain more confidence in your life's purpose and develop a meaning for it all. If you are interested in this program, book a free consult with us at beacons.ai/atherrichest to make sure we're a good fit.

Journal Prompt

1. Where, and in what people or activities, do you find your happiness and fulfilment? Write about it.
2. Write about all the things that are and aren't going well in your life right now. How can you work on the things that aren't?
3. List 10 reasons to get up in the morning and embrace what the day brings.
4. Are you your greatest supporter and friend right now? How can you be a bigger support system for yourself?
5. Write about the areas in life where you'd like to grow and evolve. Write about the areas where you're succeeding.
6. List 10 things you love the most about yourself.

Chapter 5: Owning Your Narrative

Owning your narrative is about taking control of the story of your life, shaping it in a way that reflects your values, aspirations, and experiences authentically. It begins with cultivating self-awareness, delving deep into your values, beliefs, strengths, weaknesses, and life experiences. Through this introspection, you gain a clearer understanding of how these elements have shaped your identity and the story you want to tell about yourself.

Once you have a grasp of who you are and what you stand for, it's important to define your narrative. What are the key themes, values, and messages you want to convey? This involves identifying the overarching story you want to tell about your life and the legacy you want to leave behind.

Challenging limiting beliefs is a crucial aspect of owning your narrative. Identify and challenge any negative self-perceptions or beliefs that may be holding you back from fully embracing your story. Replace these with empowering beliefs that align with the narrative you want to create for yourself.

Embracing all aspects of your journey, both the successes and the challenges, is essential. Recognize that every experience has contributed to shaping you into the person you are today and has played a role in your unique narrative.

Crafting your message involves communicating your narrative effectively through storytelling. Use language that reflects your authenticity and resonates with your audience. Share your experiences, insights, and values in a way that inspires and connects with others.

Setting boundaries is important in owning your narrative as well. Be intentional about what you share with others and how you share it. Choose how much of your personal life you want to disclose and set boundaries that align with your comfort level.
Living in alignment with your narrative means taking intentional actions that reflect your values, goals, and aspirations. Make choices that are true to yourself and live authentically in accordance with your true self.

Embracing vulnerability is a key aspect of owning your narrative. Be willing to share your authentic self, including your fears, insecurities, and imperfections. Vulnerability fosters connection and allows others to relate to your story on a deeper level.

Seeking feedback and support from trusted individuals who believe in your narrative is valuable. Surround yourself with supportive people who encourage your growth and provide insights and perspectives that contribute to the ongoing development of your narrative.

Ultimately, owning your narrative is a continuous process of self-discovery, growth, and evolution. By following these strategies, you can take ownership of your story and create a narrative that authentically reflects who you are and what you stand for.

Cultivating Resilience through Vulnerability

One day during a conversation about how I was feeling like therapy with a client wasn't going well, my friend stated. "What if she's just not open to what you're saying because she has a wall up? Sometimes when I'm about to get ready to talk to you, I have a wall up, but then I remember that I don't have to because you're understanding," "but maybe she hasn't realized that yet. You just have to approach things in a different way so that you are able to get through to her." *Hmm, I never thought about it like that...*

Lets delve a bit deeper, with what I call radiant insight.

"Radiant Insight" suggests a sense of clarity, illumination, and understanding that shines brightly. In the context of coaching, it could imply helping individuals gain deep insights into themselves, their goals, and their paths forward, thereby radiating clarity and understanding.

In the context of the self-discovery journey, "Radiant Insight" implies a profound understanding and clarity that emerges from within oneself. It suggests the ability to illuminate the depths of one's being, uncovering hidden truths, values, and aspirations.

Yet, both are required. A great coach must learn to coach, as well as be coachable, and I feel that there is no better coach than life itself. Not to say that there aren't great coaches out there, but let's be honest, sometimes the best insights come from the most unlikely, yet vulnerable situations. Vulnerability is important because vulnerability leads to the truth. We must be vulnerable with one another, but also vulnerable with ourselves.

Vulnerability requires honesty, honesty with one's self that we aren't perfect, and that we don't have to be. Life is a journey, it's a process or one big science experiment. We try things one way, oops, that didn't work, so we go back to the drawing board and try, try again, until we get it right. The ability to be honest about our shortcomings leads to improvement.

"You just have to approach things in a different way so that you are able to get through to her," she had said.

Hmm, I've never thought about that. Why have I never thought about that? I'm supposed to be the mentor here, and I'm the one receiving the advice. But it's true, and I know that it's true.
Not everyone can be coached and responds to the same type of coaching. I know this, I stress this, I live by this, how could I not see this?

But, but she said she was benefiting from it, and that I helped her. Yet she's not actually making any real progress, never does any homework or anything assigned to her, even when it's meant to benefit her, and she just ruminates and talks for hours about the same thing. She's regressing.

I must be a terrible coach, I'm a terrible coach. Definitely a terrible coach. A good coach would have noticed early on and wouldn't have spent months ignoring it. Good thing you're not her coach then, you're her therapist. You weren't ignoring it; you just didn't see it. You weren't originally trained to be a coach; you were trained to be a therapist. A good therapist is made to be unbiased and to be patient, up's and down's are normal. You thought she was getting better, she thought she was getting through it. She told you that you were helping her and empowering her to stand up for herself, and as a therapist, it's not your job to question that.

Then why is that not enough? Why do I feel so drained after sessions with her lately? Because you're expecting too much, you're expecting in general. That's not your job. As therapists, as coaches, we don't expect, we accept. Accept them for who they are, where they are in life, their journey, and their process, don't expect more of them than they are ready for. Her time will come.

Ugh, see this is why I don't want to be a therapist anymore, I wouldn't feel drained if I were a full-time coach already. Coaching clients want to change, they are tired of being complacent. They are, but sometimes they need grace and a little hand-holding as well. It's not easy to change, especially when people are used to living life a certain way for so long. That doesn't mean that you're a bad coach, a bad therapist, or a bad person. It's good that you see more out of her, just be patient until she sees it in herself as well.

As I grappled with the complexities of my role as both a therapist and a coach, I found myself drawn to a fundamental idea that underpinned my professional journey: expectations. In the world of therapy and coaching, expectations danced on the delicate tightrope between aspiration and reality, between hope and pragmatism. Reflecting on my experiences with clients, I realized that expectations were not just about the desired outcomes of sessions, or the progress markers meticulously plotted on a therapeutic roadmap.

They were the silent architects of the therapeutic alliance, shaping the very foundation upon which trust and growth were built. In every interaction, whether consciously acknowledged or silently present, expectations whispered their influence, setting the stage for the intricate dance of exploration and transformation. As I navigated the nuances of expectation management, I discovered that honoring and exploring these silent companions was as vital as any intervention or technique. Hidden within all of expectations lay the keys to unlocking resilience, fostering empowerment, and nurturing authentic self-discovery.

Now these expectations weren't anything that were set for me, but simply things that I expected for myself. The italicized words are part of the inner dialogue that I experienced relating to doubt, self-criticism and overthinking that I was consumed with. Whenever I would fail or felt like I had failed, I would blame myself, and criticize something I should/shouldn't have done. I would see something that could've changed and ruminate on it to no end. So when people say that 'you are your biggest critic' they're not lying.

I could do any little thing and if someone would call me out on it (including myself), even after I would be forgiven, I would feel undeserving of it. This was most often seen in my relationships where I would overreact and then apologize and say "maybe you should be single" or "maybe you're better off". This is not the same behavior that a narcissist or manipulator would use, I wasn't trying to make them feel bad or guilty, it was the exact opposite. I felt so bad and guilty and truly unworthy about myself for a simple mistake. I truly felt like I was hard to love and unbearable for having feelings and sometimes communicating ineffectively. Something so no normal for others, would send me into a depression fueled by self-loathing.

It wasn't until recently that I realized that all of this self-sabotage that I was doing to ruin things for myself and to tear myself down, was because I was the problem. AND A HUGE ONE! Not feeling worthy and capable of love and never feeling good enough is a huge problem. And I could look back and see that this was an issue in all of my failed relationships and even business endeavors. I put so much faith and belief in others, and none in myself.

Owning your narrative is about learning to accept who you are: the good, the bad, and the ugly. It's not saying "this is who I am and I can't change", but it's "this is how I was and I'm trying to change." It's about taking accountability for yourself. It's about learning to embrace life as a journey.

We talked a lot in the last chapter about our expectations vs standards from others, but first we need to have enough respect for ourselves, to set standards with ourselves. For me that might look like, "Okay, I'm not allowed to criticize myself just because I made a mistake one time" or "I'm not allowed to sulk in my negative feelings, I can feel bad or sad about the situation for about a day, but then I need to get over it." Another one is that "I need to celebrate my small wins."

I tell my clients all the time that people around you and attracted to you are a reflection of you. People treat you, how you treat you. So if I want to feel worthy, I can't be talking to myself like I'm less than. Yes, I'm not perfect, and have made mistakes, but there's always room for improvement.

Journal Prompt

Take a moment to reflect on your life story. What parts of your narrative have been shaped by others' opinions or expectations? How do you feel about those influences?

Now, envision yourself as the author of your own life. What would you change about the way you've told your story so far? What would you add, and what would you leave out?

Write about the power you hold to redefine your narrative moving forward. How can you step into your own truth and take full ownership of your story, free from outside judgment?

Consider the following questions as you write:

• What values and beliefs do you want to center in your story?
• What personal strengths do you want to highlight as you move forward?
• How will you handle any challenges or obstacles in your life story from this point on?

Remember, your narrative is yours to create—how will you write the next chapter?

Chapter 6: Healing from Within

On this journey to becoming a coach, I realized that it was not possible for me to be a good coach, without also coaching and working on myself. As a therapist who went through postpartum mental health struggles in the past year, I actually had no choice but to work on myself, otherwise there would be no way I was able to do my job almost a year later. I went from having a premature 28-week-old baby as my first child which was terribly traumatic which resulted in the need to heal myself. I had to get to know what I struggled with and overcome that before I ever claimed to be able to help others.

I have an entire coaching program that I am working on creating within one of my coaching businesses revolving around Finding Your Passion & Fulfilling Your Purpose, and this book is going to be about just that. Hopefully by the end of this book you've developed enough confidence to radiate and unleash your inner light. I intend to go a little bit deeper in future books about how to heal yourself and the importance of gaining mental clarity with actionable steps and thought-provoking questions.

So, I want to start off by saying where I am currently and where I want to be. I currently practice as a therapist, but I am looking to move into the sphere of being a life coach. And not just one specific life coach, but several types of coaches throughout several businesses: a confident coach with Livin' Authentically You, a business coach with Pretty Profit Pioneers, a mental health coach with Rae of Sunshine Mental Wealth, and then a women's health and wellness coach covering mindset, mental health, physical health, all of it, with EmpowerHer Transitions. In order to do this, I am in 2 coaching programs, and have become certified as a confidence coach already.

As a coach, it is not my job to heal you, that is something that you have to do yourself or with a therapist. I cannot help you until you've started to help yourself, so this chapter is going to help you get started. We are going to start off by defining inner healing, before going into what self-awareness and acceptance looks like, as well as different ways to heal.

Understanding Inner Healing

Inner healing is a profound journey that encompasses the integration of our mental, emotional, and spiritual dimensions. It is a process of self-discovery, self-acceptance, and self-transformation that leads to greater wholeness and well-being. In this chapter, we delve into the essence of inner healing, exploring its significance, principles, and practices that facilitate this transformative journey.

Inner healing is the process of addressing and resolving emotional wounds, traumas, and limiting beliefs that hinder personal growth and well-being. It involves acknowledging and integrating all aspects of our being—mind, body, and spirit—towards achieving inner harmony and resilience. This journey is essential for our overall wellness and fulfillment. By tending to our inner wounds and restoring balance within ourselves, we can experience profound healing, emotional freedom, and a deeper sense of purpose and connection in life.

Several principles guide the path of inner healing. Self-awareness is paramount—an honest exploration of our thoughts, emotions, and behaviors. Acceptance is key, embracing all parts of ourselves with compassion and non-judgment. Forgiveness is a powerful catalyst, releasing resentment and anger towards ourselves and others. Self-compassion nurtures healing, treating ourselves with kindness, understanding, and empathy.

Practices such as mindfulness and meditation help cultivate present-moment awareness and inner peace. Emotional processing through journaling or therapy allows us to explore and validate our feelings. Spiritual connection provides profound guidance and support, nurturing our sense of purpose and inner peace.

Understanding inner healing is the first step towards embarking on a transformative journey of self-discovery and personal growth. By embracing its principles and engaging in supportive practices, we cultivate greater resilience, compassion, and wholeness within ourselves, ultimately leading to a more fulfilling and authentic life.

Cultivating Self-Awareness and Acceptance

Self-awareness and acceptance form the bedrock of inner healing, allowing us to confront our truths, acknowledge our vulnerabilities, and embrace our inherent worthiness. As I've said before, we are all chosen by God for a reason, it's simply your job to do the work and discover the meaning.

Self-awareness is the cornerstone of personal growth and transformation. It empowers us to observe our thoughts, emotions, and behaviors without judgment, offering insights into our patterns, triggers, and underlying beliefs. Through self-awareness, we gain the power to make conscious choices, break free from automatic reactions, and align with our authentic selves.

Here are some strategies for creating self-awareness. Mindfulness practices, such as meditation, body scanning, and mindful breathing, anchor our awareness in the present moment, fostering clarity and insight into our inner experiences. Reflective journaling provides a safe space to explore our thoughts, emotions, and experiences, deepening our understanding of our beliefs, values, and areas for growth. Seeking feedback from trusted individuals offers valuable perspectives and insights into blind spots or patterns that we may not discern on our own.

Radical acceptance, on the other hand, invites us to embrace ourselves and our experiences as they are, without resistance or judgment. It involves acknowledging our strengths and limitations, successes and failures, joys and sorrows, with compassion and openness. Through radical acceptance, we cultivate inner peace, resilience, and a deeper sense of self-love and worthiness.

Embracing acceptance requires intentional practice. Engaging in self-compassion exercises, such as self-soothing touch or writing self-compassionate letters, nurtures warmth and acceptance towards ourselves. Inner child work enables us to connect with our past wounds and traumas, offering love, validation, and healing to our inner child. Affirmations and mantras that affirm our worthiness, resilience, and inherent value reinforce a mindset of acceptance and self-love.

Integrating self-awareness and acceptance into daily life involves incorporating mindfulness practices, self-compassion exercises, and acceptance techniques into our routines. By creating moments of pause and reflection amidst life's busyness, we cultivate a gentle and non-judgmental attitude towards ourselves and our experiences. Recognizing that growth and healing are ongoing processes, we embrace life with open hearts and minds, unlocking the fullness of our potential and living with greater compassion, resilience, and inner peace.

Therapeutic Techniques for Self-Healing

Therapeutic techniques for self-healing encompass a wide range of practices and approaches aimed at promoting emotional, mental, and physical well-being. While professional therapy with a trained therapist can be invaluable, there are also numerous techniques individuals can employ on their own to support their healing journey. Here are some therapeutic techniques for self-healing:

1. Mindfulness and Meditation: Mindfulness practices involve paying attention to the present moment without judgment. Meditation techniques, such as focused breathing or body scan meditation, can help reduce stress, increase self-awareness, and promote relaxation.

2. Journaling: Writing down your thoughts, feelings, and experiences in a journal can be a powerful therapeutic tool. Journaling allows you to process emotions, gain insight into patterns of behavior, and track your progress on your healing journey.

3. Self-Compassion: Practicing self-compassion involves treating yourself with kindness, understanding, and acceptance, especially during difficult times. Cultivate self-compassion by offering yourself words of encouragement, validating your emotions, and practicing self-care.

4. Creative Expression: Engaging in creative activities such as art, music, dance, or writing can be therapeutic for self-expression and emotional release. Use creativity as a means of exploring your feelings, expressing yourself authentically, and tapping into your inner wisdom.

5. Breathwork: Breathwork techniques, such as deep breathing exercises or pranayama from yoga, can help regulate the nervous system, reduce anxiety, and promote relaxation. Focus on deep, diaphragmatic breathing to calm the mind and body.

6. Visualization: Guided imagery and visualization techniques involve mentally picturing peaceful or healing scenes to evoke relaxation and positive emotions. Visualize yourself in a safe and nurturing environment, or imagine yourself overcoming challenges with strength and resilience.

7. Self-Reflection: Take time for self-reflection and introspection to explore your thoughts, feelings, and beliefs. Ask yourself open-ended questions, such as "What am I feeling right now?" or "What do I need in this moment?" to deepen your understanding of yourself.

8. Movement and Exercise: Physical activity can be therapeutic for releasing tension, boosting mood, and increasing energy levels. Find forms of movement that you enjoy, whether it's yoga, walking in nature, dancing, or participating in sports.

9. Gratitude Practice: Cultivate gratitude by focusing on the things you appreciate in your life. Keep a gratitude journal, where you write down three things you're grateful for each day, or take a moment to silently express gratitude before meals or bedtime.

10. Seeking Support: While self-healing techniques can be powerful, it's also important to reach out for support when needed. Connect with trusted friends, family members, or support groups who can offer empathy, validation, and encouragement on your healing journey.

Remember that self-healing is a process that takes time, patience, and self-compassion. Experiment with different therapeutic techniques to find what resonates most with you, and don't hesitate to seek professional guidance if needed.

Healing Through Mindfulness and Meditation: Nurturing Inner Harmony

As women, and especially as mothers, our minds are often pulled in a thousand different directions, leaving us feeling scattered, stressed, and disconnected from ourselves. In this section, we explore how mindfulness and meditation offer sanctuary amidst the chaos, guiding us back to the present moment and nurturing inner harmony and healing.

At the heart of mindfulness and meditation lies the practice of presence—the art of being fully awake and aware in the here and now. In a world dominated by distractions and constant stimulation, cultivating presence allows us to reclaim our attention and anchor ourselves in the present moment. By tuning into our breath, sensations, and surroundings, we awaken to the richness of life unfolding moment by moment.

Healing through mindfulness and meditation can be profoundly beneficial for women on their self-development journeys. These practices offer a variety of mental, emotional, and physical benefits that contribute to overall well-being.

1. Emotional Regulation and Resilience: Mindfulness teaches the skill of observing thoughts and emotions without judgment. This can help women manage stress, anxiety, and depression by fostering a sense of calm and balance. Over time, this can build emotional resilience, enabling individuals to handle life's challenges with more grace and less turmoil.

2. Enhanced Self-Awareness: Both mindfulness and meditation encourage deep introspection, which can lead to greater self-awareness. This enhanced understanding of oneself can be transformative, revealing underlying patterns of thought and behavior that may be hindering personal growth. With this knowledge, women can make more informed decisions that align with their values and goals.

3. Improved Concentration and Focus: Regular meditation has been shown to increase the thickness of the prefrontal cortex, the area of the brain responsible for executive function like decision-making and attention. This can lead to better concentration and focus, which are invaluable in both personal and professional contexts.

4. Reduction in Physical Stress Symptoms: Mindfulness and meditation can also have tangible physical benefits, including reduced symptoms of stress such as high blood pressure, chronic pain, and insomnia. By lowering stress levels, these practices contribute to better overall health, which is crucial for anyone on a self-development path.

5. Greater Compassion and Empathy: Mindfulness enhances empathy and compassion, not just towards others but also towards oneself. This can lead to improved relationships and a kinder, more compassionate approach to personal challenges and failures, which is essential for true growth and development.

Incorporating mindfulness and meditation into a self-care routine doesn't have to be time-consuming or difficult. It can be as simple as spending a few minutes each day in quiet reflection, or using guided meditations to ease into the practice. Over time, these moments of stillness can lead to profound changes in how women perceive themselves and their lives, paving the way for a richer, more fulfilling personal journey.

Journal Prompt

Healing from within involves nurturing your emotional, mental, and spiritual well-being. It's a journey of self-discovery, acceptance, and growth. Use this journal prompt to explore your inner healing process and identify ways to foster deeper self-care and healing:

1. Identifying Wounds: Reflect on any emotional or psychological wounds you may carry. What past experiences or traumas do you feel still impact you today? Write about how these experiences have affected you.

2. Acknowledging Emotions: Consider the emotions associated with these wounds. What feelings come up when you think about these past experiences? Allow yourself to fully acknowledge and express these emotions in your writing.

3. Self-Compassion: How do you currently practice self-compassion? What are some ways you can be kinder and more understanding toward yourself as you navigate your healing journey?

4. Support Systems: Who are the people in your life that support your healing? Reflect on the role of friends, family, or professionals who help you feel safe and supported. How can you lean on them more effectively?

5. Healing Practices: What practices or activities have you found helpful in your healing process? This could include therapy, meditation, journaling, exercise, or any other activities that promote well-being. How can you incorporate these more regularly into your life?

7. Letting Go: Are there any thoughts, behaviors, or relationships that you need to let go of to further your healing? What steps can you take to release these and create space for growth and positivity?

8. Personal Growth: How have you grown or changed as a result of your healing journey so far? Reflect on the strengths and insights you've gained. How can you continue to build on these?

9. Vision for the Future: Envision your healed self. What does a fully healed and balanced you look like? Describe your life, your mindset, and your relationships. What steps can you take today to move closer to this vision?

10. Gratitude: Practice gratitude by acknowledging the progress you've made and the support you've received. What are you grateful for in your healing journey?

11. Commitment to Healing: Make a commitment to your continued healing. Write a personal pledge to yourself, outlining your dedication to nurturing your emotional, mental, and spiritual well-being.

Chapter 7: The Reality of It All

Things are about to get real confusing and I apologize in advance, but I hope that I don't lose you. Up until this point, we have realized that it starts and ends with you and that you have to learn to love yourself; then we talked about owning your narrative and healing from within, and now we are about to get into the reality of it all which is that, who you are now is not who you want to be.

I mean duh right? No one reads a self-help book because they are happy with who they are now, there are parts of ourselves that we all want to change. That doesn't mean that you don't love yourself, it just means that you have accepted the person you are right now. In order to grow, you have to be confident enough in the process or else it won't last. That's why we had to take those first steps in the previous chapters, before we're going to get into the nitty gritty of it all. How to actually Radiate, and what does that even mean Rae?!

Radiate: Unleash Your Inner Light

We've finally come to the chapter that defines it all. This is the part of the book where the real change starts to happen. Hopefully you're more confident and have started to practice more self-love, if not, I need you to go back and reread the previous chapters, especially the stories of resilience and keep reading your narrative until you believe that you are chosen for a reason.

This book is as much about owning your narrative and rewriting your story as it about creating a new character and changing your own reality. Now I personally don't believe in manifesting (I believe in prayer and the power of the tongue), but use what works for you here. In order to create the life you want, you have to change. The life you have now, the person you are now, has to be erased. Maybe not completely, but there are parts of you that have to change in order for you to reach your dreams.

In the hustle and bustle of daily life, it's easy to lose sight of the remarkable spark that resides within each of us. We get caught up in the mundane routines, societal expectations, and the pressures of our responsibilities. Yet, deep within, there exists a radiant light waiting to be unleashed—a light that holds our true essence, our passions, and our potential.

Imagine for a moment a flickering flame, obscured by layers of doubt, fear, and conformity. This flame represents our inner light, the essence of who we are at our core. It's a beacon of authenticity, waiting to illuminate our path and guide us towards fulfillment and purpose.

But how do we tap into this inner radiance? How do we unleash the full potential of our light?

The journey to unleashing our inner light begins with embracing authenticity. This means acknowledging and honoring our true selves, without the masks or pretenses we often wear to fit in or please others. Authenticity is about owning our strengths and weaknesses, our passions and quirks, and embracing them wholeheartedly.

When we align our actions with our authentic selves, we emit a powerful energy that resonates with those around us. People are drawn to authenticity because it's genuine and relatable. It creates genuine connections and fosters trust, laying the foundation for meaningful relationships and experiences.

Along the path to radiance, it's essential to cultivate self-compassion. This means treating ourselves with the same kindness, understanding, and forgiveness that we would extend to a dear friend. Self-compassion involves embracing our imperfections and mistakes as part of the human experience, rather than berating ourselves for falling short of perfection. This is why we had to do the work that was necessary in part 1.

When we practice self-compassion, we create space for our inner light to shine more brightly. We release the burden of self-criticism and judgment, allowing ourselves to fully embrace who we are in this moment. In doing so, we free ourselves from the shackles of self-doubt and insecurity, empowering us to step into our full potential.

Our inner light is fueled by our passions and purpose— the things that ignite our souls and give our lives meaning. Nurturing our passions involves dedicating time and energy to the activities and pursuits that bring us joy and fulfillment. Whether it's painting, writing, gardening, or volunteering, engaging in activities that align with our passions nourishes our spirit and fuels our inner light.

Similarly, discovering our purpose involves reflecting on our values, interests, and strengths to identify how we can make a positive impact in the world. When we live in alignment with our purpose, we feel a deep sense of fulfillment and satisfaction, knowing that our actions are contributing to something greater than ourselves.

As we embark on the journey of self-discovery and inner growth, it's important to remember that our light is meant to be shared with the world. Each of us possesses unique gifts, talents, and perspectives that have the power to inspire, uplift, and transform those around us. This is why I created Unique TransfHERmatioms, with every woman's uniqueness in mind. We all require a different coaching program to get to where we want to be.

Sharing our light doesn't require grand gestures or fame; it can be as simple as offering a kind word, lending a helping hand, or sharing our talents with others. When we radiate our inner light outwardly, we create a ripple effect of positivity and kindness that extends far beyond ourselves.

In conclusion, unleashing our inner light is a journey of self-discovery, authenticity, and self-expression. It's about embracing who we are, nurturing our passions and purpose, and sharing our gifts with the world. As we embark on this journey, may we remember that our light has the power to illuminate the darkness, inspire others, and transform the world around us.

The Spark Within

We all get a second chance at life, every time we are able to wake up another day. God gave us free will to determine what we want to do with our life. Yet most of us choose to do nothing more than what we've been doing. Every day, we stick to the same routine, never faulting, never adding any excitement to our life. The world is vast, and there is so much left unexplored. When you live life the same way you always have, the same way your parents or other generations before you have, you dim the light within you that was meant to shine brightly. This ember, this flickering flame, is none other than the essence of our being, the radiant core that yearns to burst forth in a blaze of authenticity and purpose.

Imagine a forgotten treasure buried beneath layers of societal expectations, self-doubt, and the ceaseless chatter of everyday life. This treasure is your inner light, a beacon of brilliance waiting patiently to be unearthed and unleashed upon the world. When you never step out of the shadows, you will always wonder what could of been?

So how do I uncover this hidden gem? What would my life be like on the other side of doubt? What if I let go of my fears and limiting beliefs and did something that would actually fulfill me?

The journey to unveiling our inner light begins with a daring leap into the depths of self-discovery—a plunge into the murky waters of introspection and reflection. You have to be willing to jump into the ocean, even if you have no clue what lies ahead. Leaning into the burning urge within you to be different, and go against the grain a little bit, is the only way that we will unearth our truest selves with unwavering courage and conviction.

Yet, embracing our inner light is no easy feat. It requires a boldness of spirit, a willingness to shed the masks of conformity and reveal the raw, unfiltered essence of who we are. It is a journey of self-liberation, a rebellion against the forces that seek to dim our brilliance and confine us to a life of mediocrity.

Although scary, success is on the other side of fear. It is a journey of self-exploration and transformation, where each step taken brings us closer to who we were truly called to be, who God truly meant for us to be. Along the way, we may stumble and falter, but it is in these moments of struggle that we find our greatest strength— the resilience to rise again, stronger and more luminous than before.

Everyone's story is a lot greater when there's a little bit of drama, hurt, and pain that they have to endure. It makes the happy ending so much more meaningful.

As we embark on this grand odyssey of self-discovery, I want you to remember that we are not alone. We are surrounded by other women, kindred spirits who share in our urge for authenticity and purpose. Together, we can inspire one another, uplift one another, and bask in the collective glow of our shared brilliance. That is what this book is about, what the EmpowerHer Transitions business and any other business I've created is about.

So let's cast aside the shackles of doubt and fear, and embrace the radiant spark that lies within. By embracing our inner light, we illuminate the world around us, casting out the shadows of uncertainty and paving the way for a future fueled with possibility and promise. We give hope and a sense of purpose, not just for ourselves, but those around us.

We were all created with a purpose to serve one another with a talent that God gave us. Something we were blessed with, that only we could give the world in our own special way. Something that the world is missing and that made us exactly who/what someone needed us to be.

Are you going to live up to your true potential or at least find out what that could be for you? What if you purpose was simply to radiate authentically, radiating love and light to everyone you came across? A purpose doesn't have to be big and scary, it can actually be small, yet very beautiful and impactful.

Embracing Authenticity

Authenticity takes center stage as the protagonist in our quest for inner radiance. It's a concept both simple and profound, yet often elusive in a world that demands conformity and compliance. Embracing authenticity allows us to step into the spotlight of our true selves, shedding the layers of pretense and societal expectations to reveal the raw, unfiltered essence of who we are.

But what does it truly mean to embrace authenticity?

It's more than just being true to oneself; it's about embracing the entirety of our being—the light and the shadow, the strengths and the vulnerabilities, the triumphs and the struggles. No one is perfect or free from error except God and so until he decides to bless us with his presence on earth, authenticity is the art of owning our story, unapologetically and unabashedly, and allowing it to shape the narrative of our lives. Being authentic is what makes us human, it proves that we are still works in progress and it creates vulnerability.

But embracing authenticity is not without its challenges. It requires courage—the courage to stand firmly in our truth, even in the face of criticism or rejection. It demands vulnerability—the willingness to expose our deepest fears and insecurities, knowing that true connection can only be forged in the crucible of honesty. And it calls for self-compassion—the ability to treat ourselves with kindness and understanding, recognizing that we are all imperfect beings on a journey of self-discovery.

However, the rewards of authenticity are boundless! When we embrace our true selves, we create space for genuine connection and meaningful relationships to flourish. People are drawn to authenticity like moths to a flame, instinctively recognizing the sincerity and depth of character that radiates from within. Authenticity fosters trust, builds rapport, and forms the foundation of authentic community—a community where each member is seen, heard, and valued for who they truly are.

So how do we cultivate authenticity in our lives? It starts with a commitment to self-awareness—a willingness to explore the depths of our souls with curiosity and compassion. It involves listening to the whispers of our intuition, trusting in the wisdom of our inner guidance, and honoring the truths that resonate deep within our hearts.

Authenticity is also cultivated through intentional action—by aligning our words and deeds with our deepest values and convictions. It means saying "yes" when our hearts sing with excitement and "no" when our intuition whispers caution. It's about living in alignment with our true selves, even when it's uncomfortable or inconvenient.

Chapter 8: Transforming into HER

Now after all the hard work that we did in Part 1, some of you might be ready to put this book down and never pick it back up again. And I completely agree with you. Please do. Put this book down and go celebrate the growth that you went through by doing the work for the past 8 chapters, it was not easy. Treat yourself out and celebrate the fact that you stayed dedicated to your growth journey. Remember that growth is not linear, and Rome wasn't built in one day. Neither are any other masterpieces.

But also make sure to come back to this book at some point because we are not done growing yet. We're actually just getting started. So now that you love you and you're empowered, let's work on becoming the main character, sis.

The main character is thy apologies. that you've dreamed about being in your head. She's confident, beautiful, healthy, loving, caring, successful, a great mother, popular, friendly, well-respected, and classy. She has good boundaries, she's financially free, she's happy, she's loved, she's healed, she's just that girl, right? Or that woman, excuse me.

Really take a moment and imagine her. Get clear about who she is, what she's wearing, what perfume does she have on, who is she with (friends, family, romantically), what does she do, what are her hobbies. Spend some time brainstorming until she becomes clear as day.

This exercise builds off of discovering your true self and the exercises that we did in that chapter. Does the main character and your true self align? They should, but if they don't, how are they different? Is it realistic to expect yourself to become the woman that your main character is given your lifestyle? Why or why not? Once you've done that and had a serious reality check about what's truly possible from the main character and true self, how do they not align with who you are now? What aspects are you currently missing? It might be all of them.

I know when I started my self-development journey I was none of those things, and to be honest, I'm still a work in progress, but I'm a lot more healthy and healed when it comes to my relationships with others. Part 1 was about being confident internally and going through that internal battle between expectations and reality, but Part 2 is about perception.

Now again, I know that some of you might not care what others think, and that's perfectly fine, but the reality of it is, we don't just live in our own worlds. And perception is reality, meaning however people perceive you as is who you show up as to them, whether true or not. So if you're secure in who you are and don't care what anyone thinks, this isn't for you. If you're stuck in your ways and don't give a crap what people say about you, that's fine. But for those that want to be seen as a good person, loving, kind, and all those things I named previously, we have to make sure that we are showing up that way.

I checked in with myself by doing the Myers-Briggs personality test to see who I am most aligned with as a person. I tested as an INFJ and after sending the results to my man, he agreed that it described me to a T. That meant, how I perceived myself and how I wanted to show up in the world, aligned with how other people seen me as well. Well, at least those that matter most to me.

Not to say that I am a perfect person, because we both agreed that despite all the work I've done so far, I still have a long way to go where my attitude is concerned. When I get upset or frustrated, I come off as mean and very cold hearted, and that is NEVER my intention. It's like I'm the biggest witch, with a capital B. But again, perception is reality. So as much as I try to plead my case that I'm a nice, loving, kind-hearted person, people can't let me live down the fact that my attitude is atrocious.

It used to be something I just ignored when people commented on and I'd say, "oh well, that's just who I am, if you don't like it, that is your problem." But that's a very selfish, very crappy way of thinking and it got me nowhere. I lost a lot of good people that way, and the ones that stuck around and tolerate it, just have accepted that I'm a "mean" person and I hate that for me. They consider me the nicest-meanest person they know. Because I have the biggest heart but allow my trauma and mistrust of people to justify me being a bad person because I'll go to the end of the earth for the ones I love, but that's not me being main character Rae.

Main character Rae is Soft Girl Rae, and Soft Girl Rae is friendly, lovable, and a sweetheart. That's who I am on the inside, but Soft Girl Rae actually reflects that on the outside as well.

So I had to be willing to check myself before I wrecked myself, and my relationships, and realize that I was the problem. I was rude and entitled and definitely a brat at times. Eww, I get nauseated just thinking about it. But this was me for the past 25 years of my life. And despite having done the work to become a better person after college, I still had a pretty bad attitude and a zero tolerance for BS fueled by entitlement, until I listened to this podcast. It's Act Normal podcast with Jayda and Dess, episode 1 and they talked about giving others grace because "it's our first time here" on Earth. "It's everybody's first time here," they'd said and it clicked for me.

People are going to mess up and not always show up as the best version of themselves because they're human, just like me and we all have bad days. If I'm not perfect, why do I expect them to be? I don't know y'all, y'all just have to go listen to the podcast, and I hope it's as inspiring for y'all as it was for me, but that resonated with me and I had to tell my clients about it. I had to encourage them to practice grace not only with themselves, but with others because "it's our first time here and we're all just doing our best" I'd say.

For me, transforming into her meant learning to live by the golden rule and treat people how I wanted to be treated. It meant showing up as the woman I wanted people to see me as. It required a reality check, a truth moment with myself, and A LOT of freaking hard work.

The first part was to overcome the obstacles that prevented me from being able to trust and have faith in humanity. When you see the world as negative, you can't help but to be a negative person. And it hurt, thinking I was this amazing, healed person that my clients saw me as, so helpful and inspiring, but my loved ones knew the real me, and knew I was putting on a facade. It was like being two-faced and I didn't like that so I decided to change it.

The best part about our lives on earth is that for the most part, we all have free will. God gave us the power to control our lives, so if you don't like who you are anymore, you can change it. No one says you have to be stuck being that person.

Journal Prompt

Journal Prompt: Transforming Into My Ideal Self

Date: [Insert Date]

Introduction: Today, I'll explore who my ideal self is—the main character in my own life story that I aspire to become. This exercise will help me visualize my best qualities and the life I want to lead, setting the stage for my personal transformation.

1. Envisioning My Ideal Self:

- Describe the main character you dream of becoming. What qualities does she possess? How does she handle challenges? What are her strengths?
- What values does she hold dear? How do these values influence her actions and decisions?

2. Current vs. Ideal Self:

- In what ways do I already resemble my ideal self? Consider traits, achievements, and attitudes you currently possess that align with your ideal version.
- Where do I differ from her? Identify the areas where there is a gap between your current self and your ideal self.

3. Overcoming Obstacles:

- What obstacles does my ideal self face, and how does she overcome them? Imagine scenarios or challenges she might encounter and how she would successfully navigate them.

4. Daily Actions:

- What daily actions or habits does my ideal self practice? List specific behaviors or routines she engages in regularly that contribute to her success and well-being.

5. Steps for Transformation:

- What practical steps can I take to start transforming into my ideal self? Outline actionable steps you can begin implementing in your daily life to bridge the gap between your current self and your ideal self.

6. Letter to Myself:

- Write a letter from the perspective of your ideal self to your current self. What words of encouragement, advice, or wisdom does she have for you?

Closing Thoughts:

- How do I feel after this exercise? Reflect on any new insights gained and how you can use this vision to motivate and guide your future actions.

Embodying Main Character Energy

"Main character energy" refers to the empowering concept of viewing oneself as the protagonist of your own life story. This mindset encourages individuals to engage actively in shaping their personal narratives, asserting control and making deliberate choices rather than simply reacting to circumstances. The idea, popularized on social media, promotes a sense of empowerment, self-awareness, and intentional living.

At its core, main character energy involves proactivity and agency—taking initiative in one's life decisions and pursuing goals and dreams with purpose. This is complemented by confidence and self-belief, characteristics that enable individuals to face life's challenges with assurance and trust in their own decisions and abilities. Authenticity plays a critical role, urging individuals to remain true to their values, desires, and identities, rather than conforming to external expectations.

Resilience is another crucial element, embodying the strength to overcome setbacks and continue progressing, much like a main character who faces various obstacles but remains steadfast and learns from each experience. Adopting a narrative perspective, individuals are encouraged to see their life events as part of a larger story, where challenges add depth and successes contribute to the climax, providing meaning and context to their experiences.

Furthermore, main character energy emphasizes the importance of impact and influence, inspiring others and playing a significant role in the community, much as a central character would in any narrative. This includes embracing mindfulness and presence, engaging fully with the present moment to truly appreciate and savor life's experiences.
Continuous self-improvement is also integral, reflecting the evolution of a character throughout a story. By committing to lifelong learning and personal growth, individuals can adapt and enhance their life story, ensuring it remains dynamic and fulfilling.

Overall, embodying main character energy is about leading a life filled with purpose, growth, and fulfillment, actively participating in crafting an inspiring and meaningful personal narrative. It's a motivational approach that champions taking the reins of one's life and living with intention.

Journal Prompt: Embodying Main Character Energy in My Life

Date: [Insert Date]

Introduction: In this journal session, I will dive deeper into how I can embody the 'main character energy' in my daily life. This exercise aims to identify specific actions and changes that align with being the protagonist of my own story.

1. Self-Reflection (Think back to what you previously wrote about the main character, and go a little bit deeper):

- What aspects of my current life make me feel like I am the main character in my story? Consider moments when you feel empowered, engaged, and fully alive.
- In what situations do I feel more like a side character? Reflect on times when you feel passive or sidelined in your own life.

2. Defining Characteristics:

- What qualities do I admire in the protagonists of my favorite stories? List traits such as bravery, resilience, wisdom, or compassion.
- Which of these qualities do I already possess, and which do I need to develop further?

3. Setting the Scene:

- What does a typical day look like for me now? Describe your daily routine.
- How can I tweak my daily routine to enhance my main character energy? Think about incorporating actions that align with your core values and desired traits.

4. Supportive Cast:
  - Who are the supporting characters in my life that encourage my main character energy? Reflect on relationships that empower and uplift you.
  - How can I foster and prioritize these relationships?
5. Future Plot Points:
  - What goals or future plot points do I want to aim for? Consider short-term and long-term goals that excite you and feel integral to your story.
  - What steps can I take this week to move closer to these goals?
6. Affirmation:
  - Write an affirmation that reinforces your identity as the main character. Use this affirmation to remind yourself of your agency and importance in your life story.

Part 2:

Now that you have all the specifics about the main character version of you, you are going to spend time writing "a day in the life of my higher self". This is an idea I heard from my favorite YouTuber, Jaz Turner, that can really be used to help you visualize and affirm the dream life you've sought after. Our "Little Miss Soft Life" journal is a great companion workbook to help you think more deeply about this.

Chapter 9: Overcoming Obstacles

In today's society, despite significant strides toward gender equality, women continue to navigate a complex landscape of challenges and barriers. Before you can truly transform into the main character, you have to overcome the obstacles and do the work to figure out what is holding you back. This chapter opens by examining the current societal conditions for women, acknowledging the progress that has been made in areas such as education and employment while also highlighting persistent issues like wage disparities, underrepresentation in leadership, and societal expectations. The persistence of these challenges underscores the need for a focused discussion on how women across the globe continue to fight for equality and justice.

At the heart of this discussion is the resilience and resourcefulness that women have shown in overcoming these obstacles. This chapter aims to explore the multifaceted nature of these challenges, sharing both personal anecdotes and broader trends. Through this exploration, the chapter will not only shed light on the adversities women face but also celebrate the powerful ways in which they rise above them.

As we delve into these themes, it's important to recognize that the journey toward gender equality is far from over. The obstacles discussed here are not just hurdles to be cleared by individual women but are systemic issues that require collective action and societal change. Thus, this chapter also serves as a call to action, urging all members of society to contribute to a world where gender no longer dictates one's opportunities and rights. With a focus on overcoming obstacles, this narrative seeks to inspire, empower, and mobilize continued advocacy and support for women everywhere.

Section 1: Identifying Key Challenges

Workplace Inequality

One of the most pervasive challenges that women face today is workplace inequality. Despite significant advancements, women continue to encounter a gender pay gap across virtually all industries. This disparity is not merely a matter of economics but also reflects deeper systemic biases that hinder women's career advancement. Moreover, the glass ceiling remains a stubborn barrier, with women significantly underrepresented in executive and leadership roles. These issues are compounded for women of color, who often face intersecting biases that further limit their professional opportunities.

Harassment and Safety

Another critical area of concern for women is harassment and safety, both in physical and digital spaces. Women are disproportionately affected by sexual harassment in the workplace, a problem that extends into public spaces as well. Online, women are frequent targets of cyber harassment, including threats, stalking, and gender-based abuse. These experiences not only impact women's immediate safety but also their long-term psychological well-being and sense of security in professional and social environments.

Healthcare and Bodily Autonomy

Healthcare disparities significantly affect women, particularly in areas related to reproductive health and rights. In many regions, access to essential healthcare services is restricted, and policies often prioritize ideological agendas over scientific guidance and women's autonomy over their own bodies. This results in significant challenges for women seeking not only reproductive care but also equitable treatment for conditions that disproportionately affect them, such as autoimmune diseases and chronic pain conditions.

Socio-Cultural Expectations

Women are also tasked with navigating complex socio-cultural expectations that dictate their roles at home and in society. These expectations often place undue pressure on women to conform to idealized standards of beauty and behavior while also managing family responsibilities and professional ambitions. The balance between personal desires and societal expectations can create a double bind for women, who may face criticism or discrimination regardless of the choices they make regarding career and family.

By identifying these challenges, this section lays the groundwork for understanding the systemic nature of the obstacles women face. These are not isolated issues but are interconnected and require multifaceted strategies for change. The following sections will explore how women have navigated these challenges and offer strategies for overcoming them, aiming to empower readers to participate in these efforts toward a more equitable society.

Section 2: Personal Stories of Resilience as Mothers

The journey of motherhood comes with its unique set of challenges and obstacles. This section shares the stories of women who have navigated these difficulties with determination and resilience, offering inspiration and insights for other mothers facing similar situations.

Balancing Career and Family

First, we meet Lisa, a marketing executive and mother of two. Lisa struggled with the demands of a high-pressure job while managing her children's needs and her own expectations of motherhood. She often felt torn between her professional ambitions and her desire to be present for her family. Through careful negotiation for flexible work arrangements and open communication with her partner, Lisa found a balance that worked for her family, allowing her to thrive both at home and at work. Her story highlights the importance of workplace flexibility and supportive family structures in achieving work-life balance.

Overcoming Postpartum Depression
Next, there's Sarah, who faced severe postpartum depression following the birth of her first child. Feeling isolated and overwhelmed, Sarah initially struggled to seek help due to stigma and her own misconceptions about mental health. Her journey to recovery began when she opened up to a friend who had experienced similar issues. With professional help and the support of a compassionate community, Sarah managed to reclaim her strength and mental well-being, becoming an advocate for mental health awareness among new mothers.

Single Parenting Challenges
We also hear from Rachel, a single mother navigating the financial and emotional complexities of raising her children alone. Rachel faced numerous challenges, from financial insecurity to the overwhelming responsibility of making all parenting decisions solo. By leveraging community resources, joining support groups, and learning to manage her time and finances meticulously, Rachel not only provided for her children's needs but also built a strong, loving home environment. Her story is one of empowerment through community support and personal resilience.

Navigating Childcare and Career Growth

Finally, there's Anita, who returned to her career in healthcare after taking a break to raise her children. Anita faced significant challenges in re-entering the workforce, including gaps in her resume and shifts in industry standards. Determined to succeed, she updated her qualifications, sought out mentors in her field, and slowly rebuilt her career. Anita's persistence paid off as she regained her professional standing and set an example for her children about the value of perseverance and education.

These stories showcase not just the challenges of motherhood but also the resourceful and innovative ways in which these women have overcome them. Each narrative provides a blend of personal triumph and practical strategies, emphasizing the power of support systems, professional help, and personal determination. As we move forward, the next section will delve into broader strategies that can help mothers and families navigate and overcome the hurdles they face.

Lisa's Journey: Finding Work-Life Harmony

Lisa, a marketing executive at a leading tech firm, returned to work after the birth of her second child feeling the full weight of her dual responsibilities. With her career demanding long hours and her children needing her attention, Lisa often found herself working late nights after putting the kids to bed, sacrificing her own rest and well-being. The turning point came when she missed her daughter's school play due to an urgent work meeting, an event that left her reevaluating her priorities.

Determined to find a better balance, Lisa initiated a conversation with her employer about flexible working arrangements. She proposed a plan that included two days of remote work per week and adjusted her hours to better fit her family's schedule. To her relief, her employer was supportive, recognizing the value of accommodating working parents. With these changes, Lisa was able to attend school events, manage childcare more effectively, and maintain her productivity at work. Her experience underscores the importance of communication and negotiation in achieving work-life balance, and she has since become an advocate for parental rights in the workplace, helping to institute more family-friendly policies at her company.

Sarah's Battle with Postpartum Depression

After the birth of her son, Sarah found herself struggling with intense feelings of sadness, fatigue, and irritability. What she initially dismissed as normal 'baby blues' grew into overwhelming depression that made even daily tasks seem insurmountable. Ashamed and fearful of judgment, Sarah hid her struggles from family and friends until one evening, when a simple question from a close friend about her well-being brought everything spilling out.

Realizing she needed help, Sarah sought professional guidance. With the support of a therapist and joining a support group of new mothers facing similar challenges, Sarah began the slow process of recovery. Through therapy, she learned to manage her symptoms and rebuild her self-esteem, gradually regaining her sense of identity beyond motherhood. Sarah's journey led her to start a blog to share her experiences and support other mothers dealing with postpartum depression, creating a supportive community that advocates for mental health awareness in motherhood.

Rachel's Single Parenting Triumph

Rachel found herself a single mother of two after her partner abruptly left, leaving her to manage parenting and financial responsibilities alone. Initially overwhelmed, Rachel faced mounting bills and the daunting task of providing both emotional and financial support for her children. Recognizing the need for a sustainable plan, Rachel took charge of her situation by enrolling in financial literacy workshops and connecting with other single parents through community groups.

These steps not only improved her financial management skills but also provided a network of support that proved crucial. She found ways to earn a supplemental income from home and became adept at budgeting and prioritizing expenses. Rachel's resilience and proactive approach helped stabilize her family's situation, and she now leads a support group for single parents, sharing her insights and resources to empower others in similar situations.

Anita's Return to Healthcare

Anita's decision to pause her career in healthcare to raise her children was a difficult one, compounded by fears of falling behind in a rapidly advancing field. When she decided to return to work, she faced skepticism about the gap in her resume and her ability to re-adapt to the demanding environment. Undeterred, Anita enrolled in a series of certification courses to update her skills and volunteered at a local clinic to gain current experience.

Her commitment paid off as she slowly regained her confidence and professional acumen, eventually securing a position that acknowledged her past experience and new qualifications. Anita's journey highlights the challenges and triumphs of returning to work after a significant break, showcasing the power of determination and lifelong learning. She has since mentored other women looking to re-enter the workforce, providing guidance and encouragement based on her own experiences.

These stories of Lisa, Sarah, Rachel, and Anita illustrate the diverse challenges mothers face and the inspiring ways in which they overcome these obstacles, serving as powerful examples for others navigating similar paths.

Journal Prompt

Women often face unique challenges and obstacles in various aspects of their lives. Reflecting on these experiences can help in understanding, overcoming, and growing from them. Use this journal prompt to explore the obstacles you've encountered and how they have shaped you:

1. Identifying Obstacles: Think about the significant obstacles you have faced as a woman. These could be related to career, education, relationships, health, or societal expectations. Write about the most impactful challenges you've encountered.

2. Initial Reactions: How did you initially react to these obstacles? What emotions did you experience, and how did you cope with the immediate impact?

3. Support Systems: Reflect on the role of support systems in your life. Who were the people who supported you through these challenges? How did their support help you navigate the difficulties?

4. Overcoming Challenges: What strategies or actions did you take to overcome these obstacles? Were there any specific approaches that were particularly effective for you?

5. Lessons Learned: Consider the lessons you've learned from facing these obstacles. How have these experiences contributed to your personal growth and resilience?

6.Empowerment: In what ways have overcoming obstacles empowered you? Reflect on how these experiences have strengthened your sense of self and your ability to handle future challenges.

7.Ongoing Challenges: Are there any obstacles you are currently facing? How can you apply the lessons and strengths gained from past experiences to navigate these current challenges?8. Balancing Roles: Reflect on the various roles you juggle, such as professional, caregiver, partner, and friend. How do you balance these roles, and what challenges arise from managing them?

9. Self-Care: Consider how you practice self-care while dealing with obstacles. What are some ways you can prioritize your well-being and ensure you have the energy and resilience to face challenges.

10. Future Vision: Envision a future where you have successfully navigated your current obstacles. What does this future look like, and how do you feel in this envisioned life? What steps can you take today to move toward this vision?

Chapter 10: Understanding Your Feelings

Understanding your feelings is a crucial first step when facing interpersonal conflicts or challenges. Before you can effectively forgive someone or establish boundaries, you must first acknowledge and comprehend your own emotional responses to the situation. This self-awareness allows you to address these feelings constructively rather than letting them control or overwhelm you.

Start by identifying what you're feeling. Are you hurt, angry, regretful, disappointed, or perhaps a mix of several emotions? Allow yourself to feel these emotions without judgment. Recognizing that your feelings are valid is essential in understanding why you react in certain ways to people and events.

Once you've identified your feelings, explore their origins. What specific actions or words triggered these emotions? Understanding the root causes of your feelings can help in addressing them more effectively and prevent similar issues in the future.

Reflect on how these emotions affect your behavior and decision-making. Emotions can cloud our judgments and lead to reactions that we might regret later. By understanding your emotional triggers, you can begin to respond rather than react, paving the way for more thoughtful and deliberate actions.

Journaling can be a helpful tool in this process. Writing down your thoughts and feelings can provide clarity and help in tracking your emotional triggers over time. This practice not only aids in emotional regulation but also enhances self-understanding, which is invaluable when navigating complex interpersonal dynamics.

Understanding Forgiveness

Understanding forgiveness more deeply involves recognizing its complex and multifaceted nature. Forgiveness is a process that can vary significantly from person to person and situation to situation. Here are some key aspects to consider to gain a better understanding of forgiveness:

Forgiveness as a Personal Choice
Forgiveness is, fundamentally, a personal choice. It's a decision to let go of resentment and thoughts of retribution, regardless of whether the person who wronged you deserves it or has asked for forgiveness. This choice is primarily for the forgiver's peace of mind and emotional health, rather than a gift to the offender.

Forgiveness as a personal choice is a crucial aspect of the forgiveness process. It emphasizes the individual's autonomy in deciding to release negative emotions related to someone else's actions, irrespective of external pressures or expectations.

Autonomy in Forgiveness

When forgiveness is viewed as a personal choice, it becomes an act of personal empowerment. This perspective places the decision squarely in the hands of the person who has been wronged, giving them control over how to respond to the hurt. It's about choosing a path that aligns with one's values and needs, rather than being swayed by societal expectations or the desires of others.

Not Contingent on Apology

A significant aspect of viewing forgiveness as a personal choice is the understanding that forgiveness does not need to be contingent on the offender's apology or remorse. While receiving an apology can facilitate the forgiveness process, making forgiveness a personal choice means that it is possible even without an apology. This approach can be particularly empowering in situations where the offender may never acknowledge their wrongdoing or no longer be accessible (e.g., they have passed away or are completely out of contact).

Benefits of Viewing Forgiveness as a Choice

Forgiving someone can lead to numerous psychological benefits, including reduced stress and anxiety, lower levels of depression, and improved mental health. Physiologically, forgiveness can lead to lower blood pressure, improved heart health, and better immune function. Socially, it can strengthen relationships if both parties are invested in reconciliation and mutual understanding.

- Emotional Control: By choosing to forgive, individuals take control of their emotional well-being. This decision can help reduce feelings of victimhood and increase feelings of personal strength.
- Health Benefits: Numerous studies have shown that forgiveness can lead to better mental and physical health. Choosing to forgive can lower stress levels, reduce risk of depression, and even improve heart health.
- Moving Forward: Forgiveness allows individuals to move on with their lives. Holding onto anger and resentment can keep a person stuck in the past. Forgiveness, by contrast, opens up a space for future growth and new experiences.

The Process of Forgiveness

Forgiveness is often described as a process, not a single act. This process includes several stages:

1. Acknowledgement of Hurt: Recognizing and accepting that you have been hurt is the first step. Denial of hurt can delay the forgiveness process.

2. Empathy: Sometimes, trying to understand the perspective and motivations of the person who hurt you can aid in the process of forgiveness. Empathy doesn't excuse the behavior but can help in reducing personal bitterness.

3. Forgiving Yourself: At times, forgiveness also involves forgiving yourself for allowing yourself to be hurt or for the negative feelings you've harbored.

4. The Decision to Forgive: Choosing to forgive involves actively deciding to let go of resentment and other negative emotions associated with the grievance.

Challenges in Forgiving

Forgiveness can be challenging, particularly when the hurt is deep or the offender hasn't expressed remorse. Here, forgiveness can feel like it undermines justice or condones bad behavior. It's important to distinguish between forgiving and forgetting, or forgiving and condoning. Forgiveness can occur even when accountability and consequences are upheld.

Making forgiveness a personal choice is not without its challenges:

1. Misconceptions: There can be misconceptions that forgiveness means forgetting the hurt or excusing unacceptable behavior. However, true forgiveness means acknowledging the pain while choosing to let go of the anger.
2. Pressure to Forgive: Sometimes, there can be social or familial pressure to forgive, which can make it feel less like a choice and more like an obligation. This pressure can complicate the emotional process and potentially lead to feelings of resentment or insincerity in the act of forgiving.

3. Internal Conflict: Choosing to forgive can sometimes lead to internal conflict, especially if part of you feels that forgiveness might betray your hurt or suffering. Balancing the desire for justice or retribution with the potential peace that comes from forgiveness can be difficult.

Emphasizing Choice in Forgiveness

To truly embrace forgiveness as a personal choice, it is important to engage in self-reflection and possibly even seek guidance through counseling or spiritual advisement. Understanding one's own values and emotional needs is key to making a choice that feels right. Additionally, it's essential to ensure that the decision to forgive is one that brings peace or closure on personal terms, rather than feeling like a forced or empty gesture.

Forgiveness as a personal choice is fundamentally about taking control of one's emotional journey and deciding independently how best to heal and move forward. This empowered approach can lead to profound personal growth and healing.

We are now going to unpack each individual emotion typically associated with forgiveness - sadness, anger, hurt, disappointment, and regret. We will talk about why each emotion exists, their function, as well as how to manage it. The steps to managing each of these emotions will mostly be similar across the board - acknowledging the emotion, reflecting on why you feel said emotion, coming to terms with what happened through some sort of coping skill, and then seeking professional help if additional assistance is needed. Yet, there's a slight variation in a few, so we're going to go through them one by one, starting with anger.

Understanding Anger

Understanding anger and recognizing why it exists are crucial steps in managing emotions effectively and improving overall mental health. Anger is a natural human emotion that can serve important functions, but it can also lead to problems if not managed properly.

Understanding Anger

Anger typically arises when we perceive a threat or injustice. It can be triggered by external events (like being treated unfairly or experiencing frustration) or internal events (like recalling a painful memory or dealing with personal problems). The emotion of anger itself is not negative; it's a normal response that can motivate us to address problems, defend ourselves or others, and make changes. Think about a time you were angry and the purpose it served.

However, the way we handle anger can have significant positive or negative consequences. It becomes problematic when it is excessive, expressed in harmful ways, or suppressed.

Why Anger Exists

1. Protective Mechanism: Anger is part of the body's 'fight or flight' response system, which prepares us to confront or escape a perceived threat. It can increase our energy and focus our attention on the threat, helping us to protect ourselves.

2. Communication Tool: Anger can signal to others that something is wrong. It communicates dissatisfaction or displeasure, potentially prompting others to reconsider their actions or negotiate a problem.

3. Catalyst for Change: Feeling angry can motivate individuals to address injustices or problems in their environment. It can inspire action towards personal or social change, encouraging people to speak out or correct wrongs.

4. Indicator of Personal Boundaries: Anger often arises when personal boundaries are violated. It serves as an indicator that something has crossed a line with our values or personal space, alerting us to the need to reinforce those boundaries.

Managing and Learning from Anger

1. Recognize Triggers: Understanding what triggers your anger is the first step in managing it. Keep a journal or reflect on situations that make you angry to identify patterns.

2. Develop Emotional Awareness: Recognize the physical and emotional signs of anger. By becoming aware of how your body and mind react, you can take steps to calm down before acting.

3. Practice Healthy Expression: Express your anger in a healthy, non-confrontational way. Use "I" statements to describe the issue and how it makes you feel, rather than blaming or criticizing others.

4. Seek Constructive Solutions: Focus on solving the issue that triggered your anger. Consider various strategies and seek input from others if needed.

5. Learn Relaxation Techniques: Techniques such as deep breathing, meditation, or progressive muscle relaxation can help calm emotional and physical reactions to anger.

6. Seek Professional Help: If anger is frequent, intense, and affects your relationships or quality of life, consider seeking help from a mental health professional.

By understanding and addressing anger constructively, you can turn it into a tool for personal growth and improved interpersonal relationships, rather than allowing it to become destructive.

Understanding Regret

Regret is a complex emotion that arises when we reflect on past actions or decisions and wish we had chosen differently. It often involves a sense of loss or missed opportunity, and can be associated with feelings of sadness, guilt, and disappointment. Understanding regret and learning how to manage it can provide important insights into our values, decisions, and how we approach life's challenges.

Understanding Regret

Regret occurs when:

- We realize a different choice might have led to a better outcome: This could be something as simple as regretting a purchase because the item was not as useful as expected, or as significant as regretting a career choice or a relationship decision.
- We feel responsible for the unfavorable outcome: Regret is closely tied to personal responsibility. It's more intense when we believe our own actions directly led to a negative result.
- We learn from the outcome: Regret often involves hindsight, recognizing in retrospect what could have been done better.

The Functions of Regret

Regret serves several important functions:

1. Learning and Future Planning: One of the primary functions of regret is to help us learn from our mistakes. By analyzing what went wrong, we can make better decisions in the future. This adaptive aspect of regret can lead to more thoughtful choices and prevent repeat errors.

2. Personal Growth: Regret can motivate personal growth by highlighting discrepancies between our actions and our values. Understanding these discrepancies can push us to align future actions more closely with our personal values and ethics.

3. Social and Emotional Development: Experiencing regret can enhance emotional intelligence. It encourages empathy and understanding, as recognizing our own faults can make us more compassionate towards others.

Managing Regret

To effectively manage and learn from regret, consider the following strategies:

1. Acknowledge and Accept: Recognize your feelings of regret without judgement. Accepting that regret is a normal part of human experience can help you deal with it more constructively.

2. Reflect on the Decision: Analyze the decision-making process that led to the regret. Were there external pressures? Did you have all the necessary information? Understanding these factors can reduce self-blame and aid in learning.

3. Make Amends If Possible: If your actions hurt others or led to negative outcomes, consider making amends. This could involve apologizing, correcting a mistake, or taking steps to ensure it doesn't happen again.

4. Focus on What You Can Change: Concentrate on aspects of your life that you can influence. Dwelling on unchangeable past decisions only prolongs distress. Instead, use the insight gained from regret to influence future decisions.

5. Seek Professional Help if Needed: If feelings of regret are overwhelming or lead to depression or anxiety, talking to a mental health professional can be beneficial. They can provide strategies to cope with these feelings constructively.

Understanding and managing regret is about learning from the past and applying those lessons to improve future actions. By doing so, regret can be transformed from a source of continual pain to a motivating force for personal and ethical growth.

Understanding Hurt

Understanding hurt involves recognizing the emotional pain that results from feeling wronged, disappointed, or let down, either by others or by circumstances. Hurt can stem from a variety of sources, including betrayal, rejection, criticism, or neglect. It's a deeply personal emotion that can vary greatly in intensity and impact, depending on the individual and the context.

What Hurt Means

Hurt often signifies:

- A violation of trust or expectation: This occurs when someone or something doesn't meet the standards or commitments expected, which can lead to a sense of betrayal or disappointment.
- Feeling undervalued or disregarded: When our feelings, desires, or needs are ignored or minimized, it can cause emotional pain, making us feel unimportant or invisible.
- Loss of connection: Hurt frequently arises in relationships when there's a disruption in the connection, whether through misunderstanding, conflict, or emotional distance.

Functions of Hurt

Hurt, while uncomfortable, serves important functions in our emotional lives:

1. Signal of Values and Boundaries: Just as physical pain alerts us to potential harm to our bodies, emotional pain can indicate that something is amiss in our interpersonal relationships or personal values. It can signal that our boundaries have been crossed or that our expectations need adjusting.

2. Opportunity for Emotional Growth: Experiencing hurt can lead to greater self-awareness and emotional depth. It can push us to reflect on our personal needs and the quality of our relationships, fostering growth and maturity.

3. Catalyst for Change: Hurt can motivate us to change how we interact with others or to seek changes in our relationships, ensuring that our needs are better met in the future.

Managing and Learning from Hurt

To manage and learn from feelings of hurt effectively, consider the following approaches:

1. Acknowledge and Validate the Emotion: Recognize that it's okay to feel hurt and that your feelings are valid. Suppressing or ignoring these feelings often only delays the healing process.

2. Reflect on the Source of Hurt: Understanding why you feel hurt is crucial. Is it due to a specific action, a pattern of behavior, or your own expectations and sensitivities? This reflection can provide insights into how to address the issue.

3. Communicate Your Feelings: If appropriate, express your feelings to the person involved. Use "I" statements to describe how you feel without placing blame, which can help in resolving misunderstandings and healing relationships.

4. Set or Adjust Boundaries: If recurrent patterns of hurt arise from specific behaviors or situations, consider setting or adjusting boundaries to protect yourself emotionally.

5. Seek Support: Talk to friends, family, or a professional about your feelings. Sharing your experiences can be cathartic and offer perspectives that help you cope.

6. Focus on Self-Care: Engage in activities that nurture your physical, emotional, and mental health. This can help restore your inner peace and resilience.

Understanding and managing hurt is not just about overcoming a negative experience, but about using it as an opportunity to deepen your understanding of yourself and your relationships, leading to healthier interactions and personal growth.

Understanding Disappointment

Understanding disappointment is crucial for managing our emotional responses to unmet expectations and lost opportunities. Disappointment occurs when our hopes, desires, or expectations are not realized, and it can range from mild letdown to profound sadness.

What Disappointment Means

Disappointment often signifies:

- Unmet Expectations: This is the core of disappointment. We feel disappointed when reality does not align with our expectations, whether those expectations are about events, outcomes, behaviors, or personal achievements.
- Perceived Loss: Disappointment can feel like a loss—the loss of what might have been if things had gone as hoped or planned.
- Reflection on Desires and Goals: It highlights our values and what we consider important or desirable. The intensity of disappointment can reflect how significant the unmet expectation was to our sense of self or our future plans.

Functions of Disappointment

Despite its negative connotations, disappointment serves several important functions:

1. Emotional and Cognitive Adjustment: Disappointment forces us to confront the reality that our expectations may have been unrealistic or that circumstances are beyond our control. This adjustment is crucial for setting more realistic future expectations.

2. Motivational Role: In some cases, disappointment can serve as a motivator to reassess our strategies or efforts and to try harder or differently next time.

3. Personal Growth: Experiencing and managing disappointment can lead to greater emotional resilience. It teaches us to cope with life's unpredictability and can deepen our empathy for others experiencing similar feelings.

Managing and Learning from Disappointment

To effectively manage and learn from disappointment, consider these strategies:

1. Acknowledge Your Feelings: Allow yourself to feel disappointed without judgment. It's okay to have disappointment after failed achievements. Acknowledging and embracing your emotions is the first step in processing them.

2. Assess and Adjust Expectations: Reflect on whether your expectations were realistic. Did you expect too much for what you were offering in the situation? Consider adjusting your expectations to align more closely with reality or with factors within your control.

3. Seek Perspective: Sometimes, discussing your disappointment with others can provide new insights or help you see the situation from a different angle. This can lessen the emotional impact.

4. Learn from the Experience: Analyze what led to the disappointment. Understanding what factors contributed to the outcome can provide valuable lessons for future endeavors.

5. Focus on What You Can Control: Shift your focus to actions and thoughts within your control. This can include planning how to overcome obstacles in the future or simply deciding how to respond emotionally to disappointments.

6. Practice Gratitude: Focusing on the aspects of your life that you are grateful for can help balance the scale of disappointment. Gratitude helps shift attention away from what's lacking to what's abundantly present.

Understanding disappointment is about recognizing its role as a natural, though painful, part of the human experience. By learning to manage it effectively, you can maintain emotional equilibrium and continue to pursue your goals with adjusted expectations and renewed vigor.

Chapter 11: Developing Boundaries

Once you have a clear understanding of your emotions and what triggers them, the next step is to set boundaries. Boundaries are essential for healthy relationships; they protect your emotional well-being and create mutual respect between parties involved.

Begin by defining what your boundaries are. What behaviors are acceptable and what are not? These boundaries can be related to how much time you spend with someone, how you are treated in conversations, and the personal space you need.

Communicate your boundaries clearly and assertively. It's important that the other person understands your limits and the consequences of crossing them. Be direct and honest in your communication, ensuring there is no ambiguity about what you expect.

Enforcing boundaries can often be challenging, especially if they are not respected. Be prepared to take action if your boundaries are violated. This might include distancing yourself from the person, seeking mediation, or in extreme cases, cutting ties completely. Remember, maintaining your boundaries is a form of self-respect and is crucial for your mental health.

Setting boundaries not only helps in managing how you interact with others but also signals to others how you expect to be treated. It's a vital step in establishing and maintaining healthy interpersonal relationships.

Boundaries are guidelines, rules, or limits that a person creates to identify reasonable, safe, and permissible ways for others to behave towards them, and how they will respond when someone steps outside those limits. Boundaries help people define their individuality, preferences, and needs. They are crucial for maintaining one's mental and emotional health, as they allow individuals to preserve their self-esteem, reduce stress, and foster healthy relationships.

Types of Boundaries

1. Physical Boundaries: Concerns your personal space, privacy, and body. It dictates who can touch you and under what circumstances.
2. Emotional Boundaries: Involves separating your emotions and responsibility for them from someone else's. It's about protecting your emotional energy by not taking on the emotions of others.
3. Time Boundaries: Relates to how you manage your time. This includes setting aside time for various aspects of life (work, leisure, relationships) and not allowing one aspect to intrude excessively into another.
4. Intellectual Boundaries: Concerns thoughts and ideas and is about respecting others' ideas and expecting the same in return.

5. Financial Boundaries: Pertains to money and possessions, determining what you are willing to share and with whom.

6. Workplace Boundaries: Relates to how you are treated at work, how you engage with colleagues, and how you manage professional demands.

Journal Prompt

Journal Entry: Reflecting on My Boundaries

1. Current Boundaries Review:
   - What boundaries have I set for myself recently? (Consider all areas: emotional, physical, professional, social, etc.)
   - How clear am I in communicating these boundaries to others?

2. Boundary Challenges:
   - What challenges have I faced with my boundaries lately? (Think about times when your boundaries were not respected or when you struggled to maintain them.)
   - How did I feel when my boundaries were pushed or ignored?
   - How did I respond to these challenges?

3. Effectiveness of Boundaries:
   - How effective are my current boundaries in protecting my well-being and respecting my needs?
   - Are there areas where my boundaries are too rigid or too lax?

4. Adjustments Needed:
   - What adjustments can I make to improve my boundaries?
   - Are there new boundaries that I need to set? (Consider areas of life that feel overwhelming or unbalanced.)

5. Action Plan:
- What specific steps will I take to communicate or enforce these boundaries? (Consider who you need to speak with and what you will say.)
- How will I handle pushback or resistance from others?

6. Reflections on Growth:
- How have I grown through the process of setting and maintaining boundaries?
- What have I learned about myself and my relationships through this process?

Closing Thoughts:
- How do I feel after reflecting on my boundaries today?
- What am I grateful for in my ability to set and maintain boundaries?

Establishing boundaries is an essential aspect of self-care and personal growth. It involves setting limits and rules for others on what is acceptable behavior towards you and how they can interact with you. Here are some practical steps on how to establish and maintain healthy boundaries:

1. Self-Reflection: Begin by understanding your own needs, values, and limits. Reflect on past experiences where you felt uncomfortable, resentful, or overwhelmed. These feelings often indicate where boundaries need to be set.

2. Define Your Boundaries: Clearly define what is acceptable and unacceptable in your interactions with others. This can range from how much personal time you need, to how you expect to be treated in relationships, and how you manage work-life balance.

3. Communicate Clearly: Once you know what your boundaries are, communicate them clearly, assertively, and respectfully to others. Use "I" statements to express how you feel and what you expect, without blaming or criticizing others. For example, say "I need to have some quiet time in the evenings to recharge," rather than "You're always bothering me at night."

4. Be Consistent: Consistency is key to maintaining boundaries. Enforce your boundaries every time they are tested, and do not make exceptions unless you truly feel it is appropriate. This helps others learn what you expect and respect your limits.

5. Handle Pushback Gracefully: Not everyone will respond positively when you set boundaries. Be prepared for some resistance, and handle it calmly and firmly. Reiterate your needs without getting drawn into an argument. Remember, it's not about getting approval from others, but about respecting your own needs.

6. Practice Self-Care: Setting boundaries can be emotionally draining, especially if you're not used to standing up for yourself. Make sure to take care of your emotional and physical health during this process.

7. Seek Support: If you find it difficult to set or maintain boundaries, consider seeking support from friends, family, or a professional. They can provide encouragement and offer advice on how to assert yourself effectively.

Establishing boundaries is not about isolating yourself but about building healthy relationships in which your needs and feelings are respected. It's an ongoing process that evolves as your life and your relationships evolve.

Journal Prompt

Journal Prompt: Defining My Boundaries

Date: [Insert Date]

Introduction: Today, I'll focus on identifying and defining my personal boundaries. Boundaries are essential for my well-being and help me maintain healthy relationships with myself and others.

1. Self-Reflection:

- What are my core values? (Consider what is most important to you in life—honesty, independence, privacy, respect, etc.)
- In what areas of my life do I feel discomfort or resentment? (These feelings can indicate where boundaries may be needed.)

2. Types of Boundaries: Think about different areas where boundaries apply and write about each one:

- Physical Boundaries: What are my comfort levels with personal space and physical touch?
- Emotional Boundaries: How much of my emotional life am I willing to share, and with whom?
- Time Boundaries: How do I prefer to spend my time, and what limits do I need to set to respect this?
- Intellectual Boundaries: How do I handle disagreements or discussions about beliefs and ideas?
- Financial Boundaries: What are my rules regarding lending money or sharing financial resources?
- Workplace Boundaries: What do I need to ensure I feel respected and productive at work?

3. Articulating Boundaries:
- How can I clearly define these boundaries to myself and others? (Think about specific phrases or rules you can establish.)
- What are examples of boundary violations I've experienced, and how did I feel about them?

4. Communicating Boundaries:
- How comfortable do I feel communicating my boundaries?
- What strategies can I use to effectively communicate my boundaries to others?

5. Upholding Boundaries:
- What challenges have I faced or might I face in maintaining these boundaries?
- What steps can I take to consistently enforce my boundaries?

6. Reflection:
- How do I feel after outlining these boundaries?
- What can I learn from this exercise about my needs and how to protect them?

Closing Thoughts:
- Write a commitment to yourself about respecting and maintaining these boundaries.

Communicating Boundaries

Communicating newfound boundaries effectively is crucial for maintaining healthy relationships and ensuring your own well-being. The key to doing so lies in being clear, assertive, and respectful. Here's a guide on how to approach this communication, along with a specific example.

How to Communicate Boundaries
1. Choose the Right Time and Place: Find a calm and private setting to discuss your boundaries. This ensures both parties are comfortable and can focus on the conversation without distractions.
2. Be Clear and Specific: Clearly articulate what your boundary is, why it is important to you, and how you expect it to be respected. Avoid vague statements; instead, be specific about what is okay and what isn't.
3. Use "I" Statements: Communicate from your perspective without blaming or accusing the other person. This can help in reducing the other person's defensiveness. For example, say "I feel overwhelmed when I don't have any time for myself in the evenings," instead of "You take up all my time."
4. Be Firm and Kind: Stand firm on your boundaries while being respectful and kind. Acknowledge the other person's feelings and encourage a discussion if they have concerns.

5. Offer Alternatives: If applicable, suggest alternatives that respect your boundaries while considering the needs of the other person.

6. Listen Actively: After stating your boundary, give the other person a chance to respond. Listen to their perspective and address any questions or concerns they might have.

Example: Communicating a Newfound Boundary
Scenario: You've decided you need more personal time in the evenings to relax and unwind, and you need to communicate this boundary to your partner who expects to spend every evening together.
Communication:

- Choosing the Right Time and Place: "Can we talk after dinner? I have something important to discuss that I think will benefit both of us."
- Being Clear and Specific: "I've realized that I need some time to myself in the evenings to recharge. It's important for my mental health and well-being."
- Using "I" Statements: "I feel overwhelmed and drained when I don't get some quiet time alone. This isn't about not wanting to spend time with you, but about needing some space to keep myself feeling good."

- Being Firm and Kind: "I love our time together, and I value it a lot. I'm hoping we can find a balance where I can have an hour alone each evening before we do something together, like watching a movie or talking about our day."
- Offering Alternatives: "Maybe I could take time from 7 to 8 PM for myself, and then we could have our time together? What do you think about that?"
- Listening Actively: "How do you feel about this arrangement? I'm open to hearing your thoughts or any concerns you might have."

By following this approach, you clearly communicate your needs while also considering the relationship's dynamics, encouraging a supportive and understanding response. This not only helps in setting the boundary but also strengthens the mutual respect and communication within the relationship.

Journal Prompt

Journal Prompt: Reflecting on Communicating Boundaries

Date: [Insert Date]

Introduction: Today's reflection is focused on my recent experience of communicating my boundaries. This is an opportunity to understand my feelings about the interaction and to assess how effectively I communicated.

1. Preparation:

- How did I prepare to communicate my boundary?
- What thoughts and feelings did I have leading up to the conversation?

2. The Conversation:

- Describe the setting and timing of the conversation. Was it the right choice?
- What specific words or phrases did I use to express my boundary?
- How did I feel while I was communicating my boundary? (e.g., nervous, empowered, anxious)

3. Response Received:

- How did the other person respond to my boundary?
- What emotions did I observe in their reaction?
- Were there any aspects of their response that surprised me?

4. Outcome:

- Was I able to effectively communicate and enforce my boundary?
- If the boundary was challenged, how did I handle that?
- What would I do differently next time?

5. Emotional Response:
- How did I feel immediately after the conversation?
- Have my feelings changed since then? If so, how?

6. Lessons Learned:
- What have I learned about myself from this experience?
- What insights have I gained about setting and communicating boundaries in the future?

Closing Thoughts:
- What can I affirm about myself and my growth in setting boundaries?

How to Handle Pushback Gracefully

Managing pushback gracefully when enforcing boundaries is a crucial skill that helps maintain self-respect and healthy relationships. Here are some strategies to handle resistance effectively:

1. Stay Calm and Composed: When you encounter pushback, maintaining a calm demeanor helps you respond thoughtfully rather than react impulsively. Taking deep breaths or pausing before responding can give you time to collect your thoughts.

2. Reaffirm Your Boundary: Clearly and firmly reaffirm your boundary. Use simple, direct language to restate what you need. For example, "I understand you might not agree, but I need to stick to my decision about this."

3. Empathize Without Giving In: Acknowledge the other person's feelings without compromising your own boundaries. This can be done by saying something like, "I see this is frustrating for you, and I'm sorry you feel that way, but this boundary is important for my well-being."

4. Offer an Explanation (If Appropriate): Sometimes, providing a rationale for your boundary can help the other person understand your perspective better. However, remember that you are not obligated to justify your personal limits.

5. Keep the Conversation Focused: If the other person tries to derail the conversation or change the subject to argue their point, gently steer the conversation back to the boundary issue. You can say, "I understand your concern, but we need to focus on resolving this particular issue right now."

6. Propose Alternatives: If possible, offer alternatives that still respect your boundaries. This shows your willingness to find a compromise and can often help de-escalate tension. For example, if someone wants more of your time than you can give, suggest specific times you are available.

7. Set Consequences if Necessary: If the person continues to disrespect your boundaries, be prepared to set consequences. This might mean reducing contact, ending a conversation, or taking other steps to protect your boundary. Be clear about these consequences and follow through if needed.

8. Seek Support: If you consistently face pushback and it becomes overwhelming, seek support from friends, family, or a professional. They can provide advice, help you strengthen your resolve, and offer comfort.

9. Reflect and Adjust: After the interaction, reflect on how it went. Consider what worked well and what could be improved for next time. Adjust your strategies as needed based on your experiences.

Gracefully managing pushback is about balancing assertiveness with empathy, ensuring that you respect both your needs and the emotions of others.

Practice Self Care

Self-care is essential for maintaining both physical and mental health. It involves activities and practices that nurture your well-being and enhance your energy, reducing stress and improving overall happiness. Here are some effective tips for self-care:

1. Establish a Routine: Create a daily routine that includes time for work and time for yourself. Routines can provide structure and make it easier to prioritize self-care.
2. Stay Physically Active: Regular physical activity is crucial for maintaining good health. It doesn't have to be intense or long; even a short walk daily can make a difference.
3. Eat Well: Nutrition plays a significant role in how you feel. Eating a balanced diet rich in fruits, vegetables, lean proteins, and whole grains can boost your energy and mood.
4. Get Enough Sleep: Adequate sleep is vital for good health. Aim for 7-9 hours per night. Develop a relaxing bedtime routine to help you wind down and ensure a good night's sleep.

5. Practice Mindfulness and Meditation: These practices can help reduce stress and improve your emotional well-being. Spend a few minutes each day in meditation or practice mindfulness in everyday activities.

6. Limit Screen Time: Excessive time in front of screens can negatively affect your mental health. Set limits on how much time you spend on devices, especially before bed.

7. Connect with Others: Maintaining social connections can support emotional health. Spend time with friends or family, or join a club or group that interests you.

8. Pursue Hobbies: Engage in activities that you enjoy and that make you feel relaxed. Whether it's reading, gardening, painting, or playing music, hobbies can provide a great outlet for stress.

9. Practice Gratitude: Take time each day to think about things you are grateful for. Gratitude can shift your mindset from what you lack to what you have, promoting a positive mood.

10. Take Breaks: Regular breaks throughout the day can help prevent burnout. Even short pauses can refresh your mind and improve productivity.

By incorporating these self-care tips into your routine, you can improve your resilience, reduce stress, and enjoy a more balanced life.

Chapter 12: Practicing Forgiveness

Now that you have learned a lot about yourself and started to do the work and the healing that is necessary to radiate, I'm sure that you have noticed a difference in your confidence already. And that's good, but we're not done. Now that you have learned your worth and started to prove to yourself that you're worthy, we want to start to cultivate positive relationships. Not only that, but we are going to talk about how to communicate effectively so that you can stay in positive relationships.

Practicing forgiveness is a powerful way to release resentment and heal emotional wounds. Forgiveness isn't about condoning wrongdoings or forgetting the harm caused, but about letting go of the grip that past hurts have on your life. Here are steps and tips to help you practice forgiveness:

Understanding Forgiveness
We've already talked about the emotions that can occur surrounding forgiveness - hurt, regret, sadness, anger, and disappointment.

1. Recognize the Benefits: Understanding the benefits of forgiveness can motivate you to embrace the process. Forgiveness is linked to reduced anxiety, depression, and major psychiatric disorders, as well as lower levels of stress and better heart health.
2. Acknowledge the Hurt: Before you can forgive, you need to fully acknowledge the hurt that was caused. Be honest about the pain and allow yourself to feel the emotions without judgment.
3. Empathize with the Offender: Try to see the situation from the other person's perspective. Consider their motivations, circumstances, and background. This doesn't excuse their behavior but can help you understand it better.

Steps to Practice Forgiveness

1. Reflect on the Incident: Think about the event that caused your pain. Reflect on how you've reacted and how it has affected your life.
2. Decide to Forgive: Forgiveness is a choice. Decide that you want to let go of the anger and resentment. This decision might need to be made repeatedly if negative feelings re-emerge.
3. Work Through Your Emotions: Recognize and process your emotions. You might feel sadness, anger, or confusion. Processing these emotions is crucial for healing.
4. Write a Forgiveness Letter: Write a letter to the person who hurt you, detailing the hurt and your decision to forgive. You don't have to send it; this can be just for you.
5. Seek Understanding and Growth: Look for lessons and insights that can be gained from the experience. What has it taught you about resilience, boundaries, or compassion?
6. Let Go of Expectations: Release any expectations of the other person or the outcome of your forgiveness. Forgiveness is for your peace and may not change the other person or reconcile the relationship.
7. Celebrate Your Decision: Acknowledge the strength it takes to forgive. Celebrate your decision to let go and move forward, recognizing it as a pivotal step in your emotional growth.

A common theme in the previous chapter on understanding the feelings relating to forgiveness was that we had to reflect on and let go of our expectations. When you seek forgiveness using any of the 7 steps we just talked about, specifically steps 4 or 5, you will feel a release within yourself. Remember that forgiveness is not for them, it's for you, so that you can heal without holding onto that hurt, disappointment, sadness, regret, or anger.

The forgiveness letter in specific is such a therapeutic practice used by many, especially when coupled with destroying the letter in some way afterwards. Whether you burn it or rip it up after writing, you are letting go of any space that the trauma/hurt held in your heart, as well as your head. It is freeing. Something that is also helpful to remember with regard to step 6 is that "it's everyone's first time here" (on earth). Even if you believe in past lives and the spiritual realm, you've never been this you before, which means you can't possibly know what's going to happen. And you can't possibly do more than what you did in that moment. Speaking back to your most traumatic events, you couldn't have prevented whatever happened from happening, you didn't know. There was no way you could have known. Having not known, don't fault yourself for what you did or didn't do.

Ongoing Practice

- Practice Self-Forgiveness: Often, it's just as important to forgive yourself as it is to forgive others. Acknowledge mistakes you've made, learn from them, and forgive yourself.
- Incorporate Mindfulness: Mindfulness practices can help you manage and release negative emotions associated with the past. This can support your forgiveness process.
- Seek Professional Help: If you find it difficult to move past certain hurts, consider seeking the help of a therapist. They can guide you through complex emotions and facilitate your healing journey.

Practicing forgiveness is a deeply personal process that requires time and patience. It's about making peace with the past to improve your present and future well-being.

Chapter 13:
Radiating Positivity

In a world that often seems clouded by negativity and stress, learning to radiate positivity is not just a skill— it's a transformative art that reshapes our lives and the lives of those around us. This chapter, "Radiating Positivity," delves into the compelling power of a positive outlook and provides you with the tools to not only foster this mindset within yourself but also to extend its warm glow into every corner of your existence.

It's not about remaining so optimistic that you become delusional, oblivious to the dangers in the world, however, we don't want to only focus on the negatives either. It's about learning to find a balance, and embrace the changes that God requires of us. In order to get to where we want to or even need to be, we cannot be the same person we once were. That requires us to embrace change with an open-mind and an open heart. Here's how.

Embracing Change

Change is a constant in life, yet it is often met with resistance or fear. Embracing change, rather than fearing it, can open up opportunities for growth and transformation. This chapter will explore how to recognize, accept, and leverage change to enhance personal development and overall well-being.

Understanding Change

Change can manifest in various forms: a new job, a move to a different city, the beginning or end of a relationship, or even shifts in personal beliefs and attitudes. Understanding that change is a natural and inevitable part of life is the first step towards embracing it. It's important to recognize that change often brings about discomfort because it challenges our status quo, pushing us out of our comfort zones.

The Psychology of Change

Humans are creatures of habit, wired to seek consistency and predictability. However, this preference for stability can lead us to overlook the benefits of adapting to new circumstances. Embracing change requires a shift in mindset from viewing change as a disruptor to seeing it as a catalyst for growth. This mindset shift involves:

- Reframing: Viewing potential challenges as opportunities.
- Resilience: Building the emotional resilience to deal with the uncertainty that comes with change.
- Flexibility: Cultivating a flexible approach to life's twists and turns.

Steps to Embrace Change

1. Acknowledge Your Feelings: Confront any fears or anxieties about the change. Acknowledging these feelings is crucial in moving forward.
2. Seek Information: Understand the implications of the change. Gathering information can reduce uncertainties and help you feel more prepared.
3. Develop a Support System: Surround yourself with supportive people who encourage your growth. Their perspectives can also help you see the positive aspects of change.
4. Set Small, Achievable Goals: Break down the change into smaller steps. Achieving these can help build confidence and reduce the overwhelm of a larger transition.
5. Celebrate Small Wins: Recognize and celebrate each step forward. This reinforces positive feelings associated with the change.

Adapting to New Realities

Once you've begun to embrace the change, the next step is integration into your daily life. This might involve developing new routines, adopting new mindsets, or letting go of outdated beliefs. It's important to give yourself time to adjust and be patient with the process.

Transformative Outcomes

By embracing change, you open yourself up to new experiences, learning opportunities, and the potential for unexpected joy. Many find that once they start embracing change, they become more creative, proactive, and energized. They also report feeling more in control of their lives and their destinies.

Conclusion

Embracing change is not just about coping with life's transitions; it's about actively participating in your own life story. By accepting and welcoming change, you not only enhance your adaptability but also deepen your understanding of yourself and your capacities. This chapter has equipped you with strategies to not only manage but celebrate change, helping you to navigate your journey with courage and optimism.

Positivity is more than just feeling happy; it's a powerful stance that can influence every aspect of your life, from how you handle stress to how you interact with others. Radiating positivity isn't about ignoring life's challenges but about approaching them with a mindset that promotes resilience and growth. This chapter explores the transformative power of positivity and provides practical strategies to cultivate and sustain a positive outlook.

Understanding Positivity

At its core, positivity is an attitude that encourages looking for the best in situations, people, and oneself. It involves focusing on the potential for good, even in challenging circumstances, and maintaining hope and joy across different aspects of life.

The Benefits of Positivity

Research has consistently shown that positivity can enhance mental and physical health, improve relationships, and increase overall life satisfaction. Some key benefits include:

- Stress reduction: Positive emotions can help buffer the impact of stress.
- Improved health: Positivity is linked to better immune function and longer lifespan.
- Greater resilience: A positive outlook enables you to recover from setbacks more quickly.

- Enhanced relationships: Positivity makes you more approachable and helps foster stronger social connections.

Cultivating Positivity

1. Practice Gratitude: Start or end each day by reflecting on things you are grateful for. Gratitude shifts your focus from what's lacking to what's abundant.
2. Mind Your Language: The words you use can shape your perception of reality. Use positive, empowering language in your self-talk and interactions with others.
3. Surround Yourself with Positive Influences: Choose to spend time with people who uplift you and avoid those who drain your energy. Similarly, consume media that boosts your spirits rather than depletes them.
4. Engage in Activities You Love: Doing things that make you feel good can naturally enhance your mood and outlook.
5. Help Others: Acts of kindness and helping others can increase your sense of life satisfaction, enhance your mood, and foster a positive state of mind.

Handling Negativity

While cultivating positivity is beneficial, it's also important to handle negativity appropriately. This doesn't mean ignoring negative feelings or situations but rather addressing them constructively. Acknowledge your feelings, seek to understand their origins, and approach them with the intent to resolve or learn from them.

Understanding Negativity

Negativity often stems from our reactions to unexpected challenges or disappointments. It can manifest as feelings of anger, sadness, frustration, or fear. While it's a natural human emotion, unchecked negativity can lead to stress, anxiety, and a pessimistic outlook on life.

Accepting Life's Unpredictability

"Life just be life-ing" sometimes and we don't always know what to expect. Often times, despite our best efforts, good things happen to bad people without a specific rhyme or reason. Embracing this reality can reduce the impact of negative emotions and help you respond more adaptively. Here's how:

1. Expect the Unexpected: Understand that not everything will go as planned. Life's unpredictability is not a reflection of your capabilities or worth, but rather a natural part of human existence.
2. Develop Flexibility: The more you can adapt to changes and setbacks, the better you can manage negativity. Flexibility allows you to adjust your expectations and find new ways to move forward.
3. Focus on What You Can Control: When faced with challenges, concentrate on the aspects of the situation that you can influence. This might be your attitude, your effort, or your next steps.

So as a mental health professional, I occasionally work with people court ordered to do substance use treatment. Although I am not entirely familiar with the 12-steps or any of the programs related to substances, I did familiarize myself with the Serenity prayer.

It reads:

"God, grant me the serenity to accept the things I cannot change, Courage to change the things I can, And wisdom to know the difference."

This saying has become something that I use even with my therapy clients, simply because there are so many things that we get stuck on in life that prevent us from living in the moment. *Well what if I would've done this, or said that, or not done this or not said that. They treated me so badly.* And on and on and on.

The fact is that it's already done. There's no going back and changing things. So when you decide to accept the things you can't change, you are no longer holding on to what could've been. Think back to the letter of forgiveness I talked about in the previous chapter. That is a perfect example of this. And then if there are things that you can change, say some meaningful relationships, a job that you really enjoyed that you'd like another shot at, or just another chance in life in general, then you want to be able to have the courage to do that without hesitation. That's where the wisdom part of it all comes in, because you gotta know what's worth fighting for and what isn't.

That's why I'm sounding like a broken record over here when I keep saying accept and acknowledge your feelings, reflect on why it hurt you or why it mattered, practice gratitude, practice self-care, work on yourself. It's all a part of the process. It's all interconnected. The purpose of this book is to become more fulfilled and to live a more meaningful life. You cannot get there, without doing these things.

We, as women, are soft, feminine beings. Acknowledging your feelings and allowing yourself to sit with your emotions, is what makes us human. Don't shy away from that, but also don't be stuck in the rut and unwilling to change because you think you're right.

Something that I've started to have my general mental health clients do is to keep two separate jars. One is an "affirmation" jar and the other is a "doubts" or "limiting beliefs" jar. Negative thoughts are inevitable, especially when life starts to happen to us, but when we're able to reflect and remember that everything happens for a reason and everything that happens was meant to happen *for* us and not *to* us, it changes everything. So basically what you do is get two mason jars, and label both. Then you want to get post-it notes and everyday, or all at once, whichever is easiest, you're going to write out each individual doubt or affirmation on a sticky note. You're going to put the doubts in their perspective jar, and of course the affirmations in their own jar. Most people start off with more doubts than affirmations.

So then for every doubt, we have to go in and counteract that with an affirmation. So if my doubt is "I am ugly." I'm then going to crumble that up, put that in my doubts jar which is me mentally 'throwing that thought away' and then I either write out or pick from the affirmation jar.

I then say, or write that affirmation 5 times aloud in the mirror, or until I believe it. So let's say I picked out "I have a big heart." So I'd say that 5 times and then put it together.

Although I am not the prettiest girl in the world, I AM someone's dream girl, and I know I have a big heart and I accept me for me. My dream partner will accept and love me for me because I love me for me.

Ideally, we want to get to a point where we're erasing out the first part and just saying "I am someone's dream girl..." The key here is to make it believable. So if you say "I'm gorgeous" but you don't feel gorgeous, you are often times going to make yourself feel worse. Or if you say "I'm smart" but you know you aren't as educated in an area as you could be, you don't leave room for growth. But admitting that I am perfect to someone or enough for someone, will point you in the right direction.

People can struggle with affirmations alone because they don't believe what you are forcing them to say, so with you, when you're combatting the negative thoughts, make it believable.

Strategies for Managing Negativity

1. Mindfulness and Awareness: Practice mindfulness to become more aware of your thoughts and feelings without judgment. This awareness can help you notice when negativity arises and choose a constructive response.

2. Reframe Negative Thoughts: Challenge and reframe negative thoughts. For example, instead of thinking, "Everything always goes wrong," try, "Sometimes things don't go as planned, and I can handle it."

3. Cultivate Positivity: Balance negativity by cultivating positive emotions. Engage in activities that bring joy, practice gratitude, and connect with supportive people.

4. Express Emotions Constructively: Find healthy ways to express your feelings, such as talking to a friend, writing in a journal, or engaging in physical activity. Expression can prevent feelings from building up and leading to overwhelm.

5. Learn from Experiences: Use negative experiences as opportunities to learn and grow. Reflect on what you can take away from each situation to improve future outcomes.

6. Seek Professional Help: If negativity becomes overwhelming or persistent, consider seeking help from a mental health professional. Therapy can provide tools to cope with negativity and improve your outlook.

Embracing Life as It Is

Accepting that "life be life-ing" means recognizing that life is a mix of good and bad, and that's perfectly normal. It involves embracing life with all its imperfections and uncertainties, and understanding that each experience, whether positive or negative, contributes to your growth. This acceptance can lead to a more peaceful and resilient state of mind, where you are better equipped to handle whatever life throws your way.

Chapter 14: The Journey Continues

Self-development is an ongoing journey. We will never be done becoming the best versions of ourselves. The minute that we evolve, and become "our dream woman", we'll settle in and enjoy that lifestyle, until we develop a new dream or goal that we want to achieve.

This is the beauty of the human experience—we are constantly growing, changing, and setting new goals. It's what keeps life exciting and full of possibilities. As we continue on our journey of self-discovery and personal growth, it's important to remember that there is no destination. Each milestone we reach is simply a stepping stone to the next chapter in our lives.

So, embrace the journey, no matter where you are on your path. Celebrate your growth, but don't become complacent. Keep striving for more, for better, and for greater fulfillment. The journey continues, and it's up to you to make the most of it. Here are some of the steps that you could take as this book comes to an end:

1. Create a Personal Development Plan: Reflect on the insights gained from the book and create a plan for further growth. Set specific, measurable goals and outline the steps needed to achieve them.
2. Practice Daily Reflection: Set aside time each day to reflect on your thoughts, feelings, and experiences. Journaling can be a powerful tool for self-discovery and personal growth.
3. Engage in Regular Self-Care: Make self-care a priority in your daily routine. This could include activities like meditation, exercise, reading, or spending time in nature.
4. Seek Support: Build a support network of friends, family, or a mentor who can provide guidance and encouragement as you continue your journey.
5. Stay Curious and Open-Minded: Maintain a curious attitude towards life and stay open to new ideas and experiences. This will help you continue to learn and grow.
6. Practice Gratitude: Cultivate a sense of gratitude for the blessings in your life. Regularly take time to appreciate the positive aspects of your life.

7. Set Boundaries: Establish healthy boundaries in your relationships and commitments. Learn to say no to things that drain your energy or don't align with your values.

8. Seek Growth Opportunities: Look for ways to continue learning and growing, whether through classes, workshops, or seeking out new experiences.

9. Celebrate Your Progress: Acknowledge and celebrate your achievements, no matter how small. This will help you stay motivated and inspired on your journey.

10. Stay Connected: Stay connected with the principles and teachings of the book. Revisit key chapters or passages regularly to reinforce your commitment to personal growth.

To reach out to Unique TransferHerMations and schedule a free discovery session, readers can visit our website at www.uniquetransfhermations.com. On our website, they can find more information about our coaching programs, services, and how we can support them on their journey of self-discovery and personal growth.

Your light is meant to shine—don't keep it hidden any longer. Radiate: Unleash Your Inner Light is your invitation to step into your power, embrace your purpose, and live a life of intention and joy.

Don't wait for the perfect moment to begin.
Start your journey today and discover the brilliance that's been inside you all along.

Are you ready to radiate? Grab your copy now and take the first step toward the life you deserve.

To schedule a free discovery session, readers can fill out a contact form on our website or send us an email at contact@uniqueytransfhermations.com. In the email, they can briefly introduce themselves, share their goals or challenges, and indicate their availability for a session.

During the discovery session, readers will have the opportunity to speak with one of our experienced coaches, who will listen to their needs, provide guidance and support, and discuss how our coaching programs can help them achieve their goals. The discovery session is a great way for readers to learn more about our approach and determine if our services are the right fit for them.

We look forward to connecting with readers and supporting them on their journey of empowerment and transformation!

Thank you for making it to the end of this book! We wish you the best!

www.ingramcontent.com/pod-product-compliance
Lightning Source LLC
Chambersburg PA
CBHW071717120626
46550CB00001B/269